# The Book of Exercise and Yoga for Those with Osteoporosis

## A Program of Movement and Meditation for Better Bones, Balance, and Posture
### 2nd Edition

Copyright © 2011 by Living Well Yoga and Fitness.
All rights reserved. No part of this publication may be reproduced or transmitted in any form or by any means, electronic, mechanical, including photocopy, recording, or any other information storage and retrieval system, without the prior written permission of the publisher.

ISBN number: 9781453707623

Produced by:
Living Well Yoga and Fitness.
www.lwyf.org

# Acknowledgments

My sincere gratitude to my students living with osteoporosis. For showing up for class at the crack of dawn in all kinds of weather with a smile, a winning attitude, and a willingness to share your experiences, support, and friendship to all who come to class. You are, and will continue to be, an inspiration to us all.

# Dedication

This book is dedicated to the more than 44 million people affected by osteoporosis and their families. Proceeds from the sale of this book will be donated to help find a cure.

# Preface

## Using Movement and Meditation To Manage Osteoporosis

*"All glory comes from daring to begin."*

- Charles Lindburgh

## What is Osteoporosis

  Osteoporosis, is a condition in which the bones become weak. Having osteoporosis means that the bones become thin, porous and fragile and are more likely to break. When a bone is weakened by osteoporosis, the spongy portion of the bone grows larger and develops more holes which weaken the internal structure of the bone. While any bone can be affected, it is most common in the bones of the hip, spine, and wrist. A hip fracture often requires hospitalization and in some cases major surgery and it can impair a person's ability to walk unassisted. Spinal fractures can cause loss of height and severe back pain. Both may lead to prolonged or permanent disability and even death.

  Bone is not a hard and unchangeable structure, in fact your bones are made of living, growing tissue. Throughout life they go through a continuous process of breaking down old bone and replacing it with new bone. The skeletal system replaces itself about every seven years. Since bones are constantly changing they can heal and be affected by diet and exercise.

| Normal Bone | Bone affected by Osteoporosis |
|---|---|

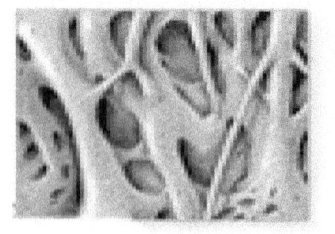

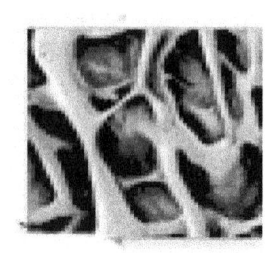

# Who Gets Osteoporosis

Osteoporosis is a major national health concern. The cost of treating it is approximately $17 billion a year ($47 million each day) and the cost is rising. Current estimates indicate that approximately 44 million Americans, or 55 percent of people 50 years of age and older are at risk for osteoporosis. While women are four times more likely than men to develop the disease, men can also be affected. Of the 10 million Americans estimated to have osteoporosis, eight million are women and two million are men. Osteoporosis is not just an older person's disease it can affect children, teenagers and young adults who are sedentary and do not get enough calcium.

The following factors may increase the chances of developing osteoporosis.

- *Age.* After maximum bone density and strength is reached which is around age 30, bone mass begins to naturally decline.
- *Gender.* Women over 50 have the greatest risk of developing osteoporosis; in fact, women are four times more likely than men to develop it.
- *Race.* Caucasian and Asian women are most likely to develop osteoporosis. Hip fractures are twice as likely to occur in Caucasian women as in African American women.
- *Bone structure and body weight.* Women and men who are thin or have smaller frames have a greater risk of developing osteoporosis, in part because they have less bone to lose than those with greater body weight and larger frames.
- *Personal history of fracture after age 50.*
- *Family history.* Heredity is an important risk factor for osteoporosis. If your parents or grandparents had osteoporosis or suffered a fractured hip after a minor fall, you may be at greater risk of developing the disease.
- *Estrogen deficiency* as a result of menopause, especially when it occurs early or is surgically induced.
- *Low testosterone levels in men.*
- *Amenorrhea* or abnormal absence of menstrual periods
- *History of eating disorders* such as anorexia nervosa.
- *Inadequate calcium intake*
- *Use of certain medications*, such as corticosteroids and anticonvulsants.
- *An inactive lifestyle.*
- *Cigarette smoking.*
- *Excessive use of alcohol.*

# Signs and Symptoms

Osteoporosis is often referred to as a "silent disease" because bone loss can occur without symptoms. People may not know that they have osteoporosis until their bones become so weak that a sudden strain, bump, twist or fall causes a fracture. However, as the disease progresses, some of the symptoms listed below may develop.

- Back pain due to fractures or postural changes.
- Loss of height.
- Stooped posture or a curved upper back (dowager's hump). Vertebrae which are the bones of the spine that are weakened by osteoporosis, may become thin and break and collapse on top of each other. This is called a compression fracture. Having collapsed vertebrae in any part of the spine results in a loss of height.
- Fractures.
  - One in two women and one in four men over age 50 will experience an osteoporosis-related fracture. Osteoporosis is responsible for more than 1.5 million fractures annually, including approximately 300,000 hip fractures, 700,000 vertebral fractures, 250,000 wrist fractures, and 300,000 fractures at other sites.
  - An average of 24 percent of those aged 50 and over who fracture a hip die in the year following their fracture. The rate of hip fractures is two to three times higher in women than men, however the risk of death one year after a hip fracture is nearly twice as high for men as for women.
  - A woman's risk of hip fracture is equal to her combined risk of breast, uterine and ovarian cancer.
  - One-fourth of those who were ambulatory before their hip fracture require long-term care afterward.
  - At six months after a hip fracture, only 15 percent of hip fracture patients can walk across a room unaided.
  - More than 90 percent of hip fractures are associated with osteoporosis.
  - Nine out of ten hip fractures in older Americans are the result of a fall.

# Prevention and Treatment

The following are steps that can optimize bone health and help prevent osteoporosis.
- A balanced diet rich in calcium and vitamin D.
- Regular participation in weight-bearing exercise.
- A healthy lifestyle with no smoking or excessive alcohol intake.
- Regular bone density testing.
- Medication when appropriate.

*Bone Density Testing*

It is important to get regular bone mineral density (BMD) tests which are also called a DEXA scans. DEXA stands for "dual-energy x-ray absorptiometry." While standard x-rays show changes in bone density after about 40 percent of bone loss, a DEXA scan can detect changes after about a one percent change. This test is non-invasive and painless and it can identify osteoporosis, determine your risk for fractures and monitor your progress when receiving treatment for osteoporosis. Your results are compared to two norms, "young normal" and "age-matched." Young normal, known as your T-score, compares your bone density to optimal or peak density of a 30 year old healthy adult. Age-matched, known as your Z-score, compares your bone density to what is expected in someone of your age and body size. Among older adults low bone density is common, so comparison with age-matched norms can be misleading.

The difference between your bone density and that of a healthy young adult is referred to as a standard deviation (SD). According to the World Health Organization individuals whose T-score is within one standard deviation of the "norm" are considered to have normal bone density. The test results are given in numbers identifying the level of osteoporosis you have.

*World Health Organization definitions of osteoporosis based on bone density levels:*
Bone density score of higher than –1 is considered normal
Bone density score of -1 to -2.5 is considered low bone density or osteopenia
Bone density score of more than -2.5 is considered osteoporosis.
Bone density score of more than -2.5 along with one or more osteoporotic fractures is considered severe osteoporosis.

The National Osteoporosis Foundation's *Physician's Guide to Prevention and Treatment of Osteoporosis,* suggests bone density testing for the following postmenopausal women.
- Those with one or more additional risk factors for osteoporosis besides menopause.
- Those who have had a fracture. A bone density test is recommended to determine if osteoporosis is the underlying cause of the fracture.
- Those who are 65 and older regardless of other risk factors.
- Those who have been on hormone replacement therapy for prolonged periods.

# Treatment

Treatment is aimed at managing the symptoms, working to maintain independent function, and as much as possible reducing disability from the disease. Treatment can include medication, surgery, and healthy lifestyle habits, including daily exercise.

*Medication*

Currently there are several options for medication to help slow the progression of the disease and to help rebuild bone mass. It is best to talk with your doctor or healthcare provider to determine which if any medication is appropriate for your individual situation. The National Osteoporosis Foundation (listed in the resources section of this book) has explanations of medications currently being used.

*Diet:*

Getting the right amounts of calcium and vitamin D and avoiding those habits that can negatively affect the strength of your bones is important. Calcium is a mineral your body requires for healthy bones, teeth, and overall functioning. Because your body cannot produce calcium itself, you must obtain it through foods, beverages and supplements. Studies have shown that not getting enough calcium is associated with low bone mass and an increased risk of fracture. Your need for calcium changes over your lifetime. Postmenopausal women and older men need more calcium. Your body becomes less efficient at absorbing calcium as you age, so it's important that you consume enough to offset this change.

**General Calcium and Vitamin D Recommendations.**
**Please consult with a physician or registered dietician for individual needs.**

| *Children & Adolescents* | Calcium (Daily) | Vitamin D (Daily) |
|---|---|---|
| 1 through 3 years | 500 mg | 400 IU |
| 4 through 8 years | 800 mg | 400 IU |
| 9 through 18 years | 1,300 mg | 400 IU |
| *Adult Women & Men* | Calcium (Daily | Vitamin D3 (Daily) |
| 19 through 49 years | 1,000 mg | 400-800 IU |
| 50 years and over | 1,200 mg | 800-1000 IU |
| *Pregnant & Breastfeeding Women* | Calcium (Daily) | Vitamin D (Daily) |
| 18 years and under | 1,300 mg | 400-800 IU |
| 19 years and over | 1,000 mg | 400-800 IU |

Food remains the best source of calcium over supplements especially dairy products like milk, yogurt, and cheese. However, it is also important to not consume too much calcium as that can lead to its own health problems.

In addition, there are substances that can interfere with the body's ability to use calcium. This includes foods with with high amounts of oxalate and phytate which reduce the absorption of calcium. Foods that are high in oxalate and phytate include blackberries, blueberries, raspberries, strawberries, spinach, rhubarb, sweet potatoes, berry juices, coffee, cola, almonds, chocolate, cocoa, peanuts, peanut butter, bran and wheat cereals, nuts, oats, rice and many others. While these foods are an important part of an overall healthy diet, they are not the best choices for calcium. A high salt meal an high protein intake can also hinder your body's ability to absorb calcium.

*Supplements*
Calcium supplements can come as calcium carbonate or calcium citrate and these forms vary in the amount of actual (elemental) calcium they contain. For example, calcium carbonate is 40 percent elemental calcium and calcium citrate contains 20 percent elemental calcium. To help determine how much elemental calcium is in a food or supplement read the label and look for the percent daily value or percent per serving. If the percent daily value is 50 add a 0 to the 50. For this supplement you will get 500 mg of elemental calcium per serving. In addition, you may find that you tolerate one form better than the other. Calcium is usually better tolerated if it is taken in small doses throughout the day. Chewable and liquid supplements tend to be absorbed better.

If you are concerned about your diet check with a local Registered Dietician (RD) who can help you make food and supplement choices suitable for your unique situation and lifestyle.

*Exercise.*
Exercise makes bones and muscles stronger and helps prevent bone loss. It also helps you stay active and mobile. Weight-bearing exercises are the best for preventing and managing osteoporosis. Weight-bearing exercises are activities that make your muscles and bones bear your weight and work against gravity. In addition, strength training and balance exercises can help you avoid falls and decrease your chances of breaking a bone. Bone is living tissue that responds to exercise by becoming stronger. Just as a muscle gets stronger and bigger the more you use it, a bone becomes stronger and denser when you place demands on it. When you are inactive your bones do not receive any messages that they need to be strong. Thus, a lack of exercise particularly as you get older, may contribute to lower bone mass or density.

### The difference between weight bearing and weight training exercise:

While these 2 terms are often used interchangeably they are actually very different types of exercises.

*Weight bearing exercise:*
Weight-bearing exercises done at least four to five times a week for 30 minutes each time, are the best ones for managing osteoporosis. Weight-bearing exercises are activities that make your bones bear your weight and work against gravity. Walking, hiking, stair climbing or dancing are all weight-bearing exercises that help build strong bones in the legs. Activities such as tennis, and pushups (either on the floor or against the wall) are weight bearing exercises that help to build strong bones in the wrists and arms. Yoga can also provide weight bearing exercise for both the legs and arms. Activities such as swimming, water aerobics and bicycling are not weight-bearing since your body is not working to support your weight.

Weight bearing exercises work because bones are constantly tearing down and rebuilding themselves. There are two types of cells; osteoclasts and osteoblasts that are responsible for bone growth. Osteoclasts break down bone, and osteoblasts build it up. As you perform activities that make your bones hold you up, you stimulate the growth of osteoclasts. In other words you stimulate your body to lay down more bone which strengthens them.

*Weight training exercise.*
Weight training exercises also known as strength training exercises, are activities in which you move your body through its full range of motion against some kind of resistance, such as free weights, machines, tubing or your own body weight. Weight training exercises also place demands on the bone but they mainly work to increase muscle strength. As the muscles become stronger, certain tasks such as standing, walking, rising from a chair, climbing stairs, and lifting objects becomes easier. Stronger muscles also support you during movement, decreasing your chances of losing your balance and falling.

The program in this book is an invitation to explore various types of movement and meditation as ways to manage osteoporosis. The following chapters outline the program I have been teaching to my students with osteoporosis.

Each chapter explains and illustrates various types of activity. You are not expected to do every exercise or movement in this book every day. Each chapter will examine different components of an exercise regimen, and explain how to develop an appropriate exercise routine. The resource section includes sample workout logs and routines to help you create the program that best fits your needs.

In addition, your level of fitness may be different then other readers. If you have been exercising for some time you can go a little harder or longer. If just starting out go easy and let yourself build up gradually.

Living with a chronic disease is often accompanied by feelings of losing control of one's life, being separated from activities that once brought joy and by fear of the unknown. Yet research suggests that movement therapies and one's state of mind can affect how osteoporosis expresses itself in the body. The techniques in this book can help you to gain back some sense of control over your disease and manage the symptoms of osteoporosis. Exercise alone can not cure osteoporosis, but in the long run it can help to improve everyday functioning and help you to feel less victimized by your condition. We hope you find this program helpful. Please know that you are in our thoughts and our hearts as you continue on your journey.

# Note:

This book is provided as a helpful reference source only. It is not intended as a medical guide, or a guide for self-treatment. The suggestions herein are not intended to replace appropriate medical care. If you are concerned about your health or diagnosis, seek competent medical attention. This book offers techniques that may be helpful for those with osteoporosis. If you are living with another medical condition some of the suggestions in this book may not be appropriate for you. Check with your healthcare provider about participating in this program or any other exercise class.

Never exercise to the point of pain or strain, and discontinue exercising immediately if you experience pain or pressure in the chest, dizziness, nausea, extreme muscle soreness or a worsening of symptoms. If you should experience any of the above, consult your health care provider immediately.

# Table of Contents

**Acknowledgments and Dedication** ……………………………………...……… 3

**Preface**………………………………………………………………………..4

**Introduction**
Making Exercise a Part of Your Day ……………………………….. 14

**Chapter 1**
Posture and Body Mechanics ………..…………………………………... 16

**Chapter 2**
Diaphragmatic Breathing and Aerobic Exercise.. ..…………………………... 45

**Chapter 3**
Strength Training…………………….. ………………………………… 86

**Chapter 4**
Yoga and Tai Chi for Flexibility and Balance ..………………………………121

**Chapter 5**
Relaxation Techniques and Stress Management ………………………....212

**Resource Section** ……………………………………………..……228
Sample workout logs and dairies
Sample routines
Helpful websites

# Introduction
## Making Exercise a Part of Your Day

*"Every day is a new beginning. Treat it that way.
Stay away from what might have been, and look at what can be."*
- Marsha Petrie Sue

The benefits of regular exercise have been well documented. Hardly a day goes by when we are not reminded of its importance through news broadcasts, newspapers, and magazine articles. Regular exercise combined with other healthy lifestyle choices can help you to manage your weight, lower blood pressure and cholesterol levels and reduce stress. It can also aid in the prevention and management of such conditions as diabetes, heart disease, cancer, and arthritis. While exercise can help to moderate many conditions, it is especially crucial for those who are living with a chronic disease. In the case of osteoporosis, the body is being affected by a condition that can cause a loss of mobility making everyday activities more challenging.

Activities of daily living, often called ADLs, include eating, dressing, bathing, sleeping, toileting, walking or moving about in general. Having osteoporosis can affect each of these. Some symptoms of osteoporosis (back pain, curved upper back and balance problems) may worsen over time, and can make it more difficult to do such things as getting in and out of a car, standing up from a chair, or walking.

Addressing these symptoms with regular exercise will help you manage your symptoms and allow you to remain independent. An exercise program should consist of aerobic or cardiovascular exercise, strength training exercise and stretching exercises. Regular aerobic exercise helps make the heart stronger and increases lung capacity. Aerobic exercise that is also weight bearing can improve bone strength. Strength training exercises help to increase muscular strength. Stretching exercises help maintain joint range of motion. The following chapters will explore different types of movement and discuss in detail how they can help.

Fitting exercise into your daily routine can be challenging. Below are some steps you can take to make this easier:

1) Schedule your exercise session into your day as you would a doctor's appointment or a meeting with a friend, and do not break your appointment unless it is absolutely necessary. Postponing your designated time can become a habit too easy to maintain. This could result in neglecting exercise altogether. Exercise is an important component to your overall health. Your exercise schedule should be given a priority as important as a medical appointment.

2) Schedule your exercise routine for a time of day that works best for you. This means finding a time when you feel your strongest and you know you have the time and energy to finish your routine.

3) Exercising with a partner or friend is more enjoyable then going at it alone. It keeps you motivated and on track. Making an agreement to do this is a great way to help you stick to your routine. Even if you do not feel like exercising, you may not want to let your partner down.

4) If you have time to do only part of your usual routine, do what you can. Do not skip your exercise session just because you only have time for part of it. Because unavoidable situations may occur to disrupt your routine, you may be tempted to skip exercise; a practice that too easily leads to breaking your exercise habit altogether. Missing one exercise session may tempt you to miss the next day and before long you may stop exercising altogether. By doing what you can in the time allowed helps you to maintain a rhythm of regular exercise.

5) Should you fall off track, do not be too hard on yourself. Everyone experiences periods of slipping back into old habits and routines. The important thing is that you recognize this pattern and return quickly to healthier habits and lifestyle choices. There will be times when sticking to your routine seems easy and other times when it seems like a hard chore. The longer you can stick with your regular routine the easier it will be to get back on track, if and when you falter.

6) Make a reasonable and realistic list of the reasons why you decided to start exercising and go back to it frequently. It might include such things as being able to climb the stairs more easily, put your shoes on more easily or losing ten pounds. Periodically remind yourself how staying with an exercise regimen can help improve the quality of your life.

7) Keep progress reports or workout logs of your exercise sessions. There is nothing more motivating then seeing results. Benefits can appear as early as four to eight weeks. Within this time period you may notice that some everyday activities have become easier. If you look back at your workout log you may be surprised at how many more repetitions of each exercise you can now complete or how much more aerobic activity you can tolerate. You may even have come close to accomplishing some of those goals in your list from item #6.

Remember, the most important thing is to exercise on a regular basis! Osteoporosis affects each person differently. You are the best judge of what feels right for your body. Look at other sources of exercise and movement techniques. Try various approaches. Through experimentation you will find the routine that suits your needs and helps you to accomplish your goals.

# Chapter One
## Posture and Body Mechanics

*"Success is that peace of mind that comes from knowing you've done everything in your power to become the very best you're capable of becoming."*
- John Wooden

While adhering to a regular exercise routine can help manage the symptoms of many conditions, it is equally important to be mindful of how you move your body during everyday activities. If one of your goals is to improve posture, then you should perform exercises that will strengthen and stretch the back and chest muscles in order to reach that goal. However, if you then spend the rest of your day sitting or lifting objects incorrectly, you will undo all of the benefits of your exercise session. Also, remember that incorrect posture and body mechanics can increase the chances of a fall. This chapter covers some of the basics concerning good posture and body mechanics.

First, let us examine good posture. Osteoporosis can cause many changes in the body. One of which is posture. Common postural changes include:
- A forward head position
- Rounding of the shoulders and upper back
- A forward trunk position with increased bending at the hips and knees

Some typical activities during which we may use incorrect posture include:
- Sitting and watching TV
- Working at a computer
- Driving/riding in a car
- Looking downward while reading, knitting and other activities
- Household chores
- Yard work

The following are some basic body mechanics principles to help correct posture, make everyday activities easier, and reduce the risk of falls.

- When bending, squat. Knees should be bent, back should be straight.
- Bend or hinge at the hips, not the waist. Remember to use the hip hinge motion.
- You are more steady with the feet wider apart and staggered. You are less steady with the feet closer together and parallel to each other.
- If lifting or bending compromises your balance, place your feet about hip width apart with one foot in front of the other for more stability.
- It is easier and more safe to push. It is harder and less safe to pull.
- Carry objects close to your body.
- When pushing or moving objects, use your body weight and momentum to push. Do not rely solely on arm strength.
- Lift with your legs, not your back.
- Always test the weight of the object before you try to lift it.
- Reorganize your house so that items you commonly use are within easy reach, preferably at a level between your knees and shoulders.
- Do not twist when lifting or pushing.
- When sweeping, vacuuming, shoveling, raking, etc., always face your work and move with it. Your nose, knees and toes should all be facing in the same direction.
- When performing the above mentioned activities, use a rocking motion, by transferring your weight from one leg to the other as you move. This allows your leg muscles to help with the work.

Many accidents happen in the kitchen and bathroom. Falls can happen while walking around, rising from a sitting position, and stepping out of the shower. The following are some tips for preventing falls.

- Be aware of the medications you take and their side effects. Some can increase the risk of falls.
- Try to avoid reaching out to furniture or handrails while walking. Stooping forward and reaching ahead of you can bring you out of balance and cause a fall.
- Be aware of uneven surfaces in rooms.
- Immediately wipe up any spilled liquids.
- Do not use scatter rugs that might slide on the floor. Secure them with skid-proof backing or securely tack them down. Worn or frayed rugs can cause tripping.
- If you need to use a step stool, make sure it is sturdy and secure.
- Always wear non-skid socks or slippers instead of regular socks.
- When rising from a lying down or a seated position, move slowly to avoid becoming dizzy.
- Make sure you have adequate lighting throughout the house. Use nightlights at night.
- Keep all floors clear of clutter.
- Before starting any activity, *think it through!* Make sure you place everything you need in an easy-to-get-to spot.
- Make a plan for getting help should you fall or become hurt.
- Try to locate phones throughout the house especially in areas such as the bathroom and kitchen where most accidents happen. As much as possible use cordless or cell phones you can carry with you. Make sure to place the phones at a level you can reach should you be unable to get up off the floor.
- Check in with someone on a regular basis in the event that you need help and are unable to get to a phone.
- Wear a medical alert bracelet or necklace if you fall frequently. With the push of a button, medical help will arrive quickly.

# Hip Hinge

Before examining specific activities we will learn about a movement called the hip hinge. This involves reaching the buttocks back as if you were going to sit in a chair, bending at the knees, keeping a natural arch in the low back and coming forward by bending at the hips instead of the waist.

This movement should be used when:

- Getting up and down from a chair
- Getting in and out of a car
- Lifting items off the floor and/or out of lower cabinets
- Shoveling, vacuuming, and cleaning
- Taking items in and out of an oven, washer, or dryer
- Anytime you need to stoop but cannot get down on one knee

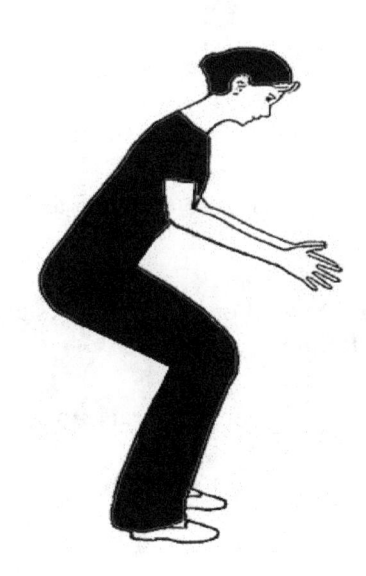

## Correct Sitting Tips

We spend much of our day sitting so it is important to learn to sit correctly.

- Avoid recliners. They promote rounding of the neck, shoulders and head and tightness in the hips.

- Avoid low, soft couches and chairs that make rising difficult.

- Choose a chair of average height with firm, smooth cushions and sturdy armrests. The height of the chair should allow for your hips and knees to be level with one another or for the hips to be slightly higher than the knees.

- Keep your chin parallel to the floor.

- Avoid crossing your legs.

- Your computer screen and TV should be at eye level to minimize neck and eye strain.

- While reading, use a book stand or rest your elbows on a pillow or table.

- A good general rule is to change your posture every 15 to 20 minutes. At this point, get up and move around.

- Chairs should have a stable base. Swivel or rocking chairs are not a good choice because they can trigger loss of balance and falling.

- To make it easier to stand up from a lower chair, raise the seat height by adding an extra cushion.

- Electric lift chairs and lift cushions can be helpful for people who have trouble getting out of chairs.

# Correct Sitting Posture

- Ears over shoulders, shoulders over hips.
- Straight back allowing for the natural curve in the low back.
- Feet flat on the floor. Shoulders are down and relaxed.
- Push the crown of the head to the ceiling, but keep your chin parallel to the floor.
- Abdominal muscles are lightly tucked in.

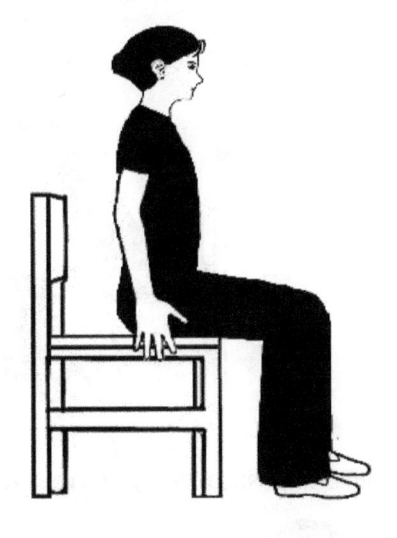

As much as you can throughout the day try to sit towards the front of the chair. This helps to avoid slouching. It also helps to strengthen the abdominal muscles as they work to hold you up. Do not sit this way for too long at first. Try sitting this way for brief periods throughout the day, (when working at the computer and at the dinner table). Slowly increase the time you sit this way each day. When you need to sit back, slide the buttocks all the way back in the chair in order to keep the ears over the shoulders and the shoulders over hips. Avoid just leaning back and slouching in the chair.

## Getting In and Out of a Chair

Falls often happen when moving from sitting to standing or standing to sitting. Protect your body and back by carefully lowering yourself in and lifting yourself out of chairs.

## Sitting to Standing

1. Bring your hips forward to the very edge of the chair (or couch) because it is more difficult to get up if you are sitting at the back of the chair.
2. Feet should be approximately shoulder-width apart or wider to provide a good base of support.
3. Position feet either parallel to each other or place your stronger leg slightly back.

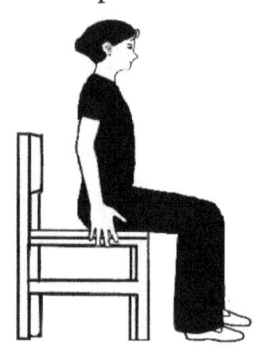

Feet parallel.

One leg slightly back.

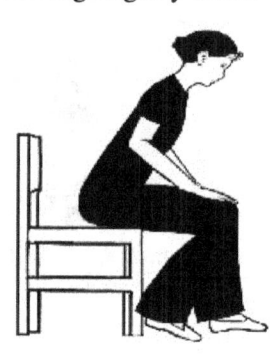

4. Lean forward at the hips until your head is positioned nose over knees and toes.

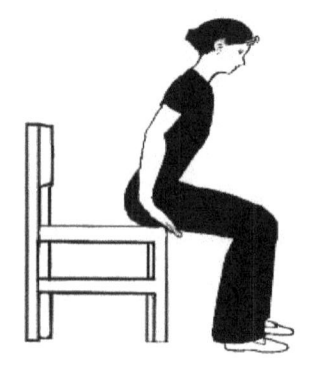

5. Continue to lean forward, bringing the nose over the toes to come up to standing. Let your legs do most of the work. Try to push off of your thighs to get up. Your leg muscles are much larger and stronger than those in your arms. If your legs are not strong enough to lift you up, you can push off the seat or arms of the chair, but avoid relying on arm strength alone to lift yourself up.

6. Keep your back straight, head up, eyes forward.

Getting up pushing off of your thighs

Getting up pushing off of the seat of the chair

Getting up pushing off of the arms of a chair

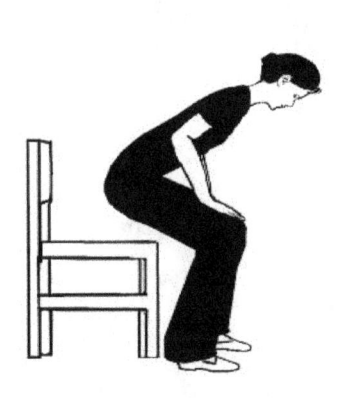

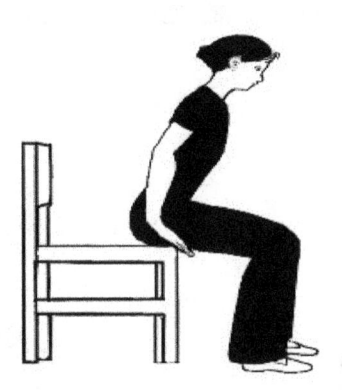

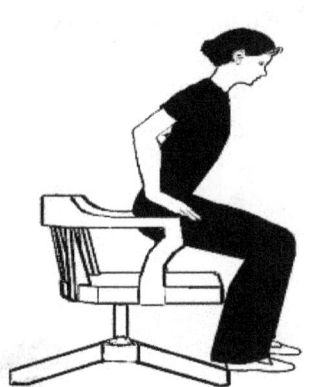

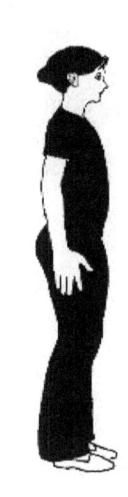

# Standing to Sitting

1. Take large rather then short shuffling steps as you approach the chair.
2. Position yourself so the chair is centered directly behind you. You should feel the chair against the back of your legs before sitting.
3. Reach back for the seat or arm rests as you "hip hinge" forward. Again think nose over knees and toes.
5. Keep your back straight, head up and eyes forward.
   *Do not turn and* reach for the chair before you sit; you might lose your balance or fall.
6. Use your leg strength to lower your body *slowly and gently* to the edge of the chair. Then slide back. If your legs are not strong enough to lower yourself to the chair, use your arms to help control your descent. *Never* crash down into a chair. Crashing down into a chair can cause injury to the back and oftentimes triggers a fall. When crashing down into a chair the chair can tip or slide out from underneath you.

Sitting down using the seat of the chair

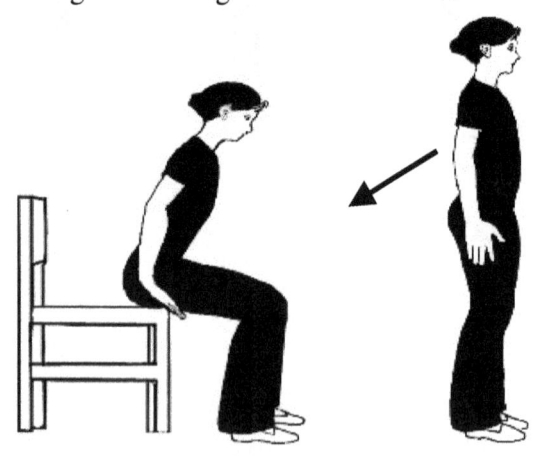

Sitting down using the arms of a chair

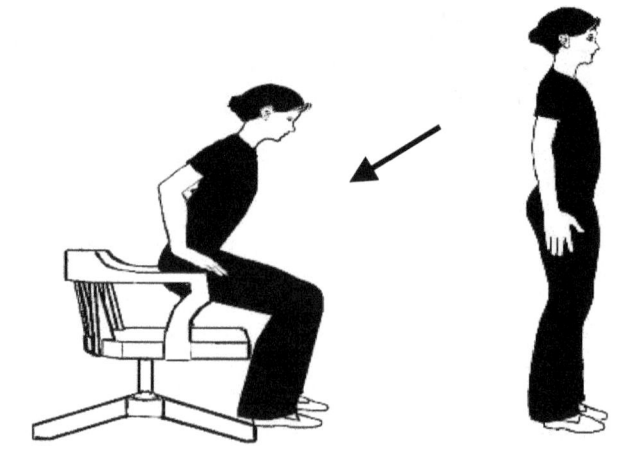

# Getting In and Out of a Car

*Avoid* stepping from a curb into a car, or from a car onto a curb. Remember always; from ground level to car, from car to ground level.

### *To get into a car*

- *Avoid* getting into a car sideways (placing one leg or foot in first).
1. Approach the car seat the same way you would a chair. Turn and back in towards the seat with your buttocks leading the way.
2. Reach back for the seat or dashboard and slowly lower yourself so you are sitting at the edge of the seat. *Never* hold on to the door which can move and trigger a fall.
3. With one hand hold onto the seat inside the car. With the other hand lift one leg at a time into the car. Then you can turn your body on the seat to face forward. Place a plastic bag on cloth seats to make turning easier.

### *To get out of a car*

- *Avoid* getting out of a car sideways.
1. Hold onto the dashboard with one hand. With the other hand, lift one leg at a time out of the car.
2. Then you can turn your body on the seat to face out.
3. Your body should be in the car and both of your legs should be out of the car and both feet flat on the ground.
4. Then, move the buttocks forward to the edge of the car seat and lean forward (hip hinge) while pushing up from the seat or dashboard. *Never* pull up on the car door, which can move and trigger a fall.

## Correct Standing Tips

- Keep your chin parallel to the floor.
- Maintain a broad base of support by keeping your feet shoulder width apart or wider.
- Abdominal muscles should be in, shoulders back and down, head and chest up and knees slightly bent, but never locked.
- An easy way to help you stand straight is to think about lifting the top of your head to the ceiling. Do not lift your chin, your chin stays parallel with the floor. As you focus on lifting the top of the head up, you may feel yourself standing taller as your abdominal and waist muscles tighten.

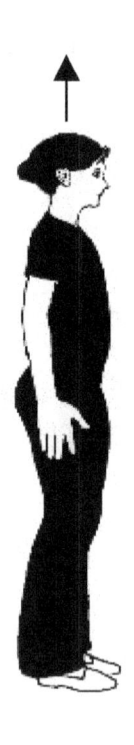

# Correct Walking

- Do not look straight down while walking. Instead look ahead and slightly down. Look down with your eyes, not your head.
- As much as possible, keep your hands free. Carry light loads in small body packs.
- If balance or strength is affecting your ability to walk, use a mobility aid such as a cane, walker or walking stick adjusted to the proper height.
- When stepping make sure you flex your front foot, letting your heel strike first. As people age they tend to shuffle; stepping on the toes first which can lead to tripping and a fall. Flexing the foot and landing with the heel first and toes up forces you to pick up your feet, lessening the risk of tripping and falling.
- When you walk make sure you swing your arms. When stepping, swing the arm that is opposite to the forward foot. Swing the arm up to shoulder height as this will aid in maintaining balance and reducing the risk of a fall.

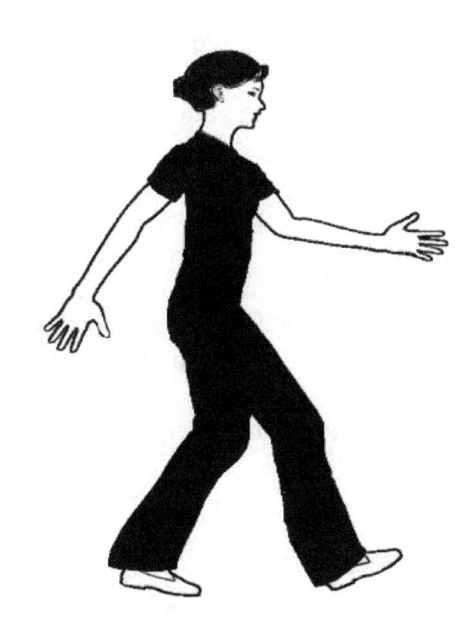

# Lying Down and Getting In and Out of Bed

It is not unusual to have trouble turning over, or getting in and out of bed. Lying on your back with a soft pillow under the knees, or on your side with a soft pillow between the knees are the best postures for sleeping. It is also good to avoid using too many pillows or too thin of a pillow under the head. Avoid sleeping in a chair. When napping lie down so that the head and neck are supported.

### *Tips for rolling or turning over in bed*
- A satin sheet or piece of satin material tucked across the middle of the bed makes it easier to turn over.
- Flannel sheets and heavy blankets can make it more difficult to turn over.
- When turning, bend your knees and put your feet flat on the bed. Allow the knees to fall to one side as you begin to roll. Turn your head in the direction you are rolling and reach the top arm across the body.
- A straight back chair anchored at the side of the bed or a bed rail can help you roll more easily.

### *Tips for scooting over in bed*
- Bend your knees placing the feet flat on the bed.
- Push into the bed with the feet and hands to lift the hips up. Then shift the hips in the desired direction.
- Finish by repositioning the feet in the direction your hips moved.

### *Helpful bedroom aids*
- A helping handle or bed rail that attaches between the mattress and box spring provides assistance with rolling and support for pushing yourself to an upright position. An inexpensive alternative to a bed rail is a straight-back chair securely laced to the bed frame.
- An adjustable blanket support keeps the blanket off feet, making it easier to move.
- A motion-activated nightlight detects movement and automatically switches on when you get up during the night to use the bathroom.
- Electric beds make it easy to elevate your head and upper body, making breathing easier.

## Getting Into Bed

1. Approach the bed as you would a chair; feel the mattress behind both legs. Reach back for the bed with your hands.
2. Slowly lower yourself to a seated position on the edge of the bed using your leg muscles to control your descent. Use the hip hinge motion (pg. 19).

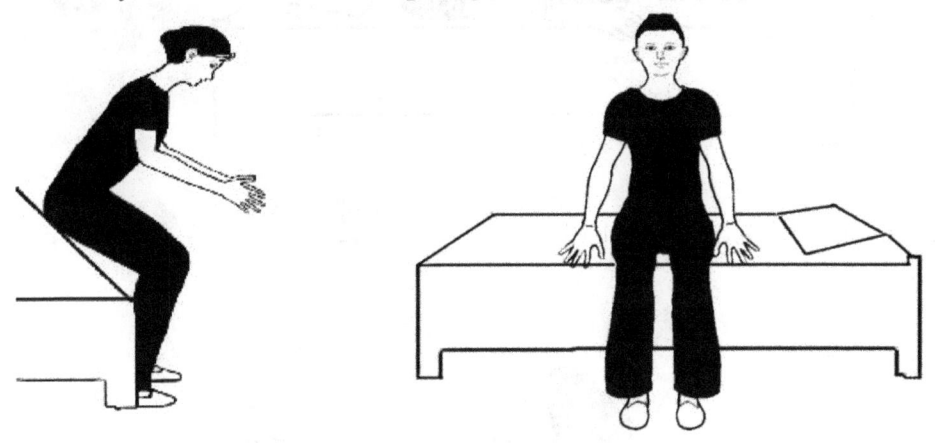

3. As your trunk goes down, bring the legs up (like a seesaw motion).

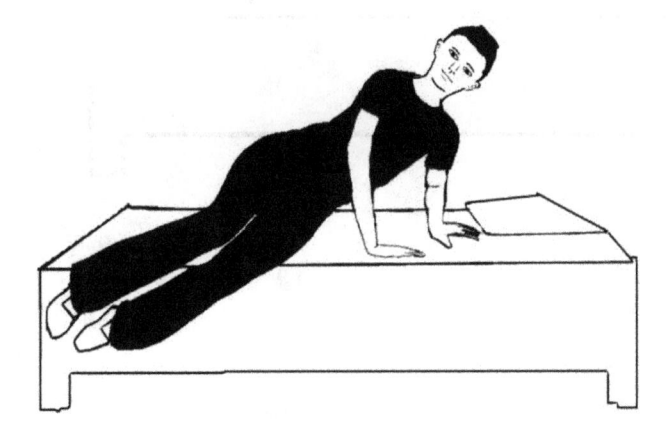

4. Use your arms to lower yourself onto your side.

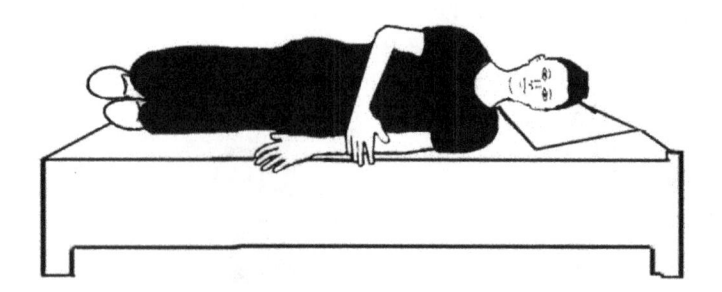

5. From here you can roll onto your back.

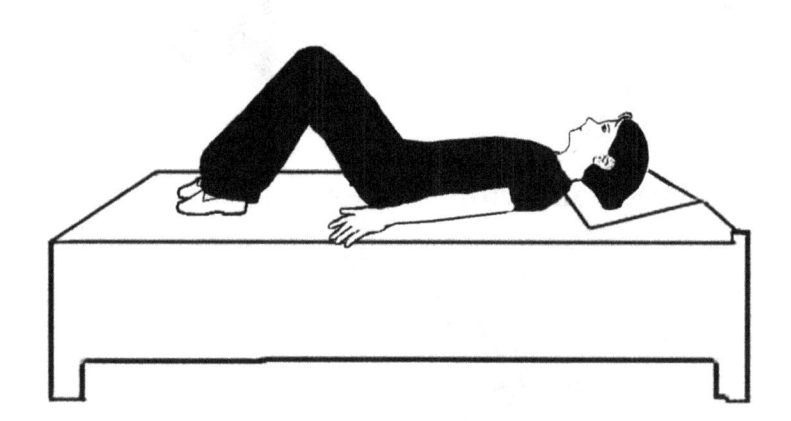

## Getting Out of Bed

Reverse the order of the above steps to get out of bed.

1. Bend the knees up and place your feet flat on the bed. Reach across with the top arm. Turn your head and look in the direction you are rolling.

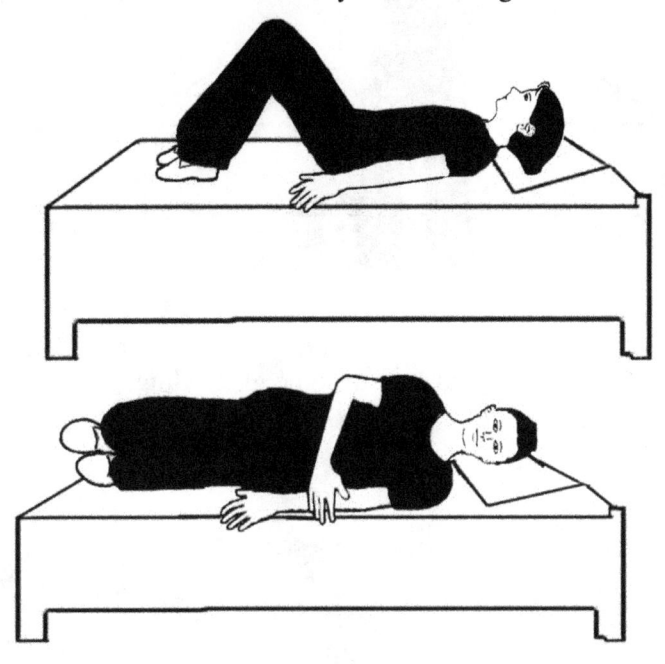

2. Roll all the way onto your side toward the edge of the bed. Let the knees fall to the side so the body moves as a unit. Push with your arms to lift the body up. As your body comes up, let the legs slide off the side of the bed.

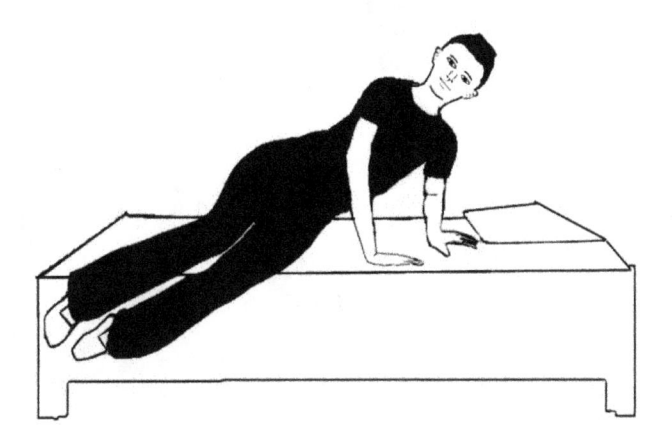

4. Lower the feet towards the floor as you push with your arms into a sitting position.

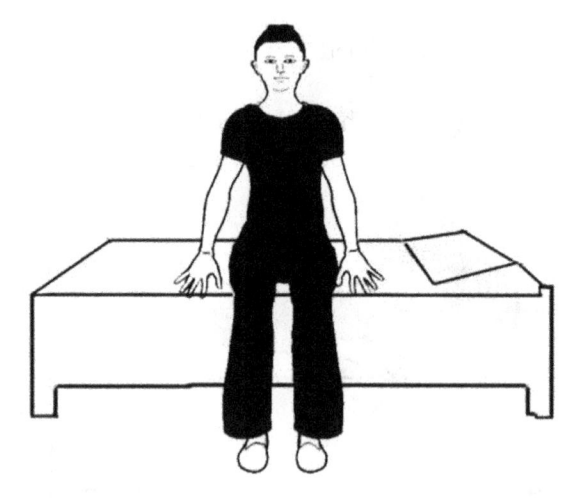

5. Slide to the edge of the bed and use your legs to come to standing. Use the hip hinge motion (pg. 19).

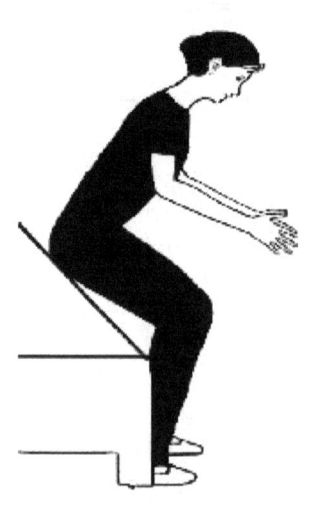

Avoid coming to a sitting position directly from your back. This strains the back muscles and is a more difficult way to get up. It is much safer to roll to your side before coming to a seated position.

# Bathing, Grooming and Toileting

## *Bathing*

Since shower stalls are easier to get into and out of than bathtubs, they are usually better for bathing. If you must use a bathtub, a tub transfer bench will help you get in and out more easily. Shower chairs allow you to sit in the shower while you bathe. Putting on a terry robe after bathing also makes drying easier.

- Bathtubs and shower stalls should have at least two grab bars to hold on to as you get in and out.
- Grab bars should always be professionally installed.
- *Avoid* using the towel bar, soap dish, or faucet as a handrail. They are not secure enough to hold your body weight.
- If you sit on a tub transfer bench or shower chair while showering, use a hand-held shower head. This will allow you to sit first and then hold the shower head to direct the water away from you so you can adjust the temperature safely.
- All bathtubs and shower stalls should have a non-skid rubber bath mat. All bath rugs should have a rubber backing.
- Be careful when using bar soap. It is slippery, hard to hold, and when dropped leaves a slippery film on the floor. Try pump soaps or soap-on-a-rope.
- Keep a nightlight on in the bathroom.
- If alone, bring a cordless or cell phone into the bathroom with you so that you can call for help if you need it. Make sure you put the phone in a place you can easily reach from the floor, should you fall.

## *Grooming*

A loss of mobility in the shoulders and upper back can make everyday tasks difficult. These tips may help.

- Sit down to brush your teeth, shave or dry your hair. Sitting not only reduces the risk of falling, but also helps conserve energy. A shower or commode chair works well for this. Leave the doors underneath the sink open to make room for your knees.
- Use a hands-free hairdryer that can be mounted on a vanity.

## *Helpful bathing and toileting aids*

- A tub transfer bench or shower chair with a back adds extra safety for those who tire easily.
- An extra-long hand-held shower spray allows you to shower while seated on a bath chair or in the tub.
- Commode frames make it easier to sit down on and get up from the toilet. Raised toilet seats also work.
- Lever faucet adapters ease grasping and turning.
- A long-handled sponge or brush helps people with limited range of motion reach the back and legs.

Remember to think about your body mechanics during all activities. For example, when brushing your teeth, try to avoid rounding the back when using the sink. Keep the back straight and bend the knees instead.

| Correct | Incorrect |
|---|---|
| Knees bent, back straight. | Knees locked, back and shoulders rounded. |

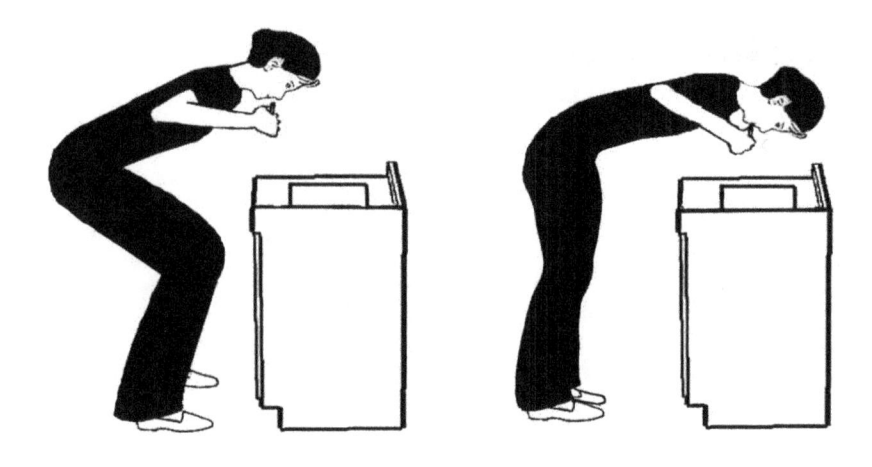

## *Dressing*

General tips for dressing

- Sit down when dressing. Choose a chair with firm support and arms. Do not sit on the edge of the bed to dress because this can lead to loss of balance and falling.
- Choose clothing with fewer buttons, zippers, and other closures that might be difficult to use.
- Replace buttons by sewing on touch fasteners such as Velcro®.
- Try loose fitting clothing made of stretchy fabric which is easy to put on.
- Bedroom slippers which can slide off your feet should be replaced with non-skid socks.
- Lightweight, supportive shoes with Velcro® closures, elastic shoelaces, or "curly fries" shoelaces make it easier to put on and take off shoes.
- An extra-long shoehorn helps shoes slide on without your having to bend over.

Remember to think about your body mechanics while dressing. For example; when putting on your shoes avoid rounding forward and either bring a foot up to your knee or put your foot on a footstool.

| Correct | Correct | Incorrect |
|---|---|---|
| Back straight, shoulders down. | Bringing your leg up instead of bending forward. | Back and shoulders rounded forward. |

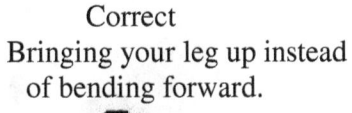

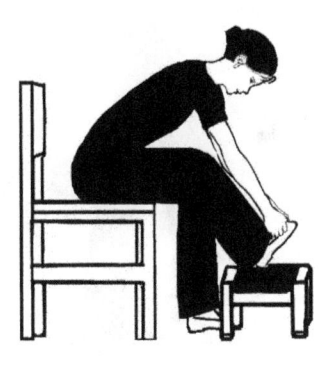

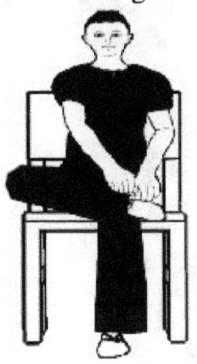

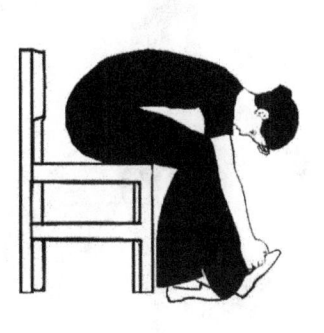

## *Household tasks*

During housework and yard work it is easy to slip into poor postural habits. Below are some guidelines to help you maintain posture and avoid falls.

- It is safer and easier to push rather than pull.
- If standing for long periods at a sink, counter, or workbench, try putting one foot up on a stool.
- When vacuuming, sweeping, or raking, always face your work. Nose, knees, and toes should all be facing in the same direction. Try to avoid twisting and bending in order to protect your back. Use a rocking motion transferring weight from one foot to the other, thereby relying on your legs to do the work instead of your back and arms.

**Correct**
Back straight; knees bent. Broom is close to body, facing work.

**Incorrect**
Back and shoulders rounded, knees locked. Broom too far away.

**Incorrect**
Twisting back and knees. Nose, knees, and toes not facing work.

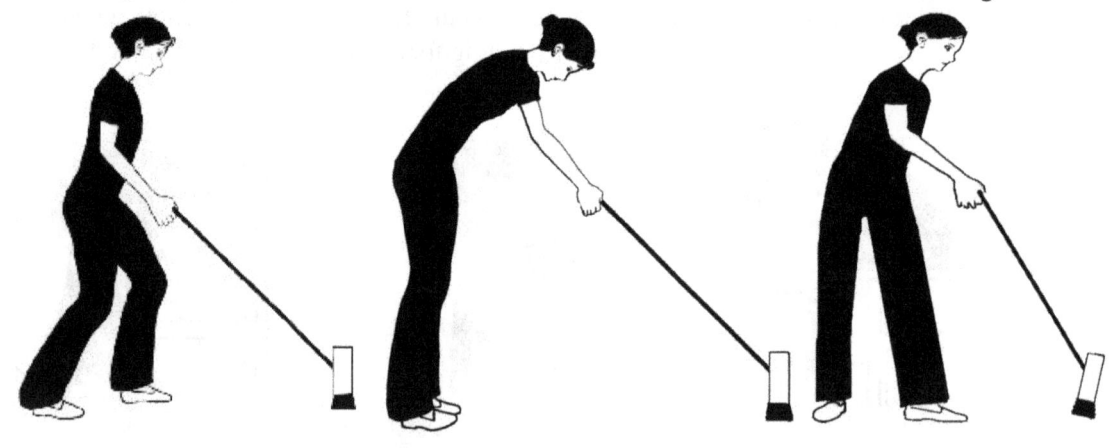

**Correct**
Correct way to sit at computer. Back straight, shoulders down.

**Incorrect**
Incorrect way to sit. Back arched screen too high

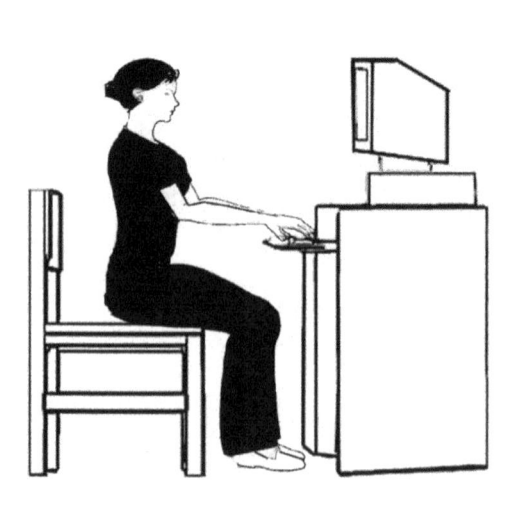

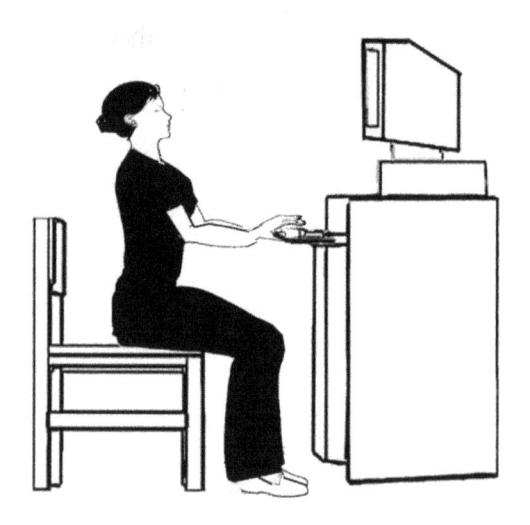

36

> When lifting always bend your knees and lift with your legs, not your back. Always test the weight of the object you are going to lift. Keep the object close to your body, and again face your work. Remember to use the hip hinge (pg. 19). Instead of rounding through the back, bend the knees, and reach the buttocks back (as if you were about to sit in a chair). Feet can be about hip width apart or wider if needed for balance. Use this motion regardless of how heavy or light the object is. Many back injuries occur just by moving the wrong way or when lifting light objects. This is especially critical if you have osteoporosis because the bones of the spine are more frail. Compression fractures can occur just by bending the wrong way and while picking up light objects.

**Correct**
Back straight, bending at hips. Stand close to the object and use your legs to lift.

**Incorrect**
Back rounded, bending at waist. Object too far away, using back to lift.

**Correct**
Correct way to carry. Keep item close to your body.

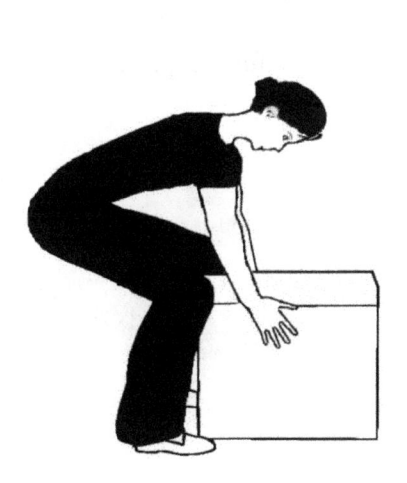

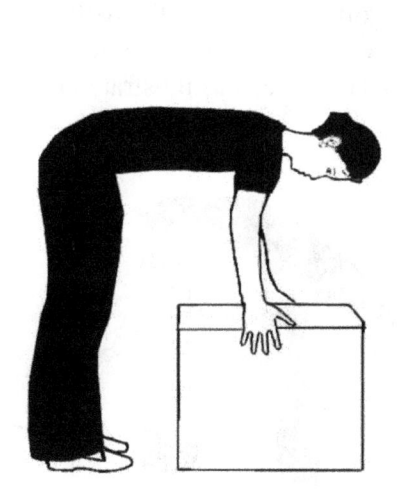

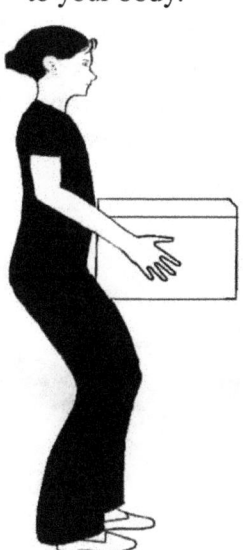

Correct way to reach items in low places. Get down and close to the object.

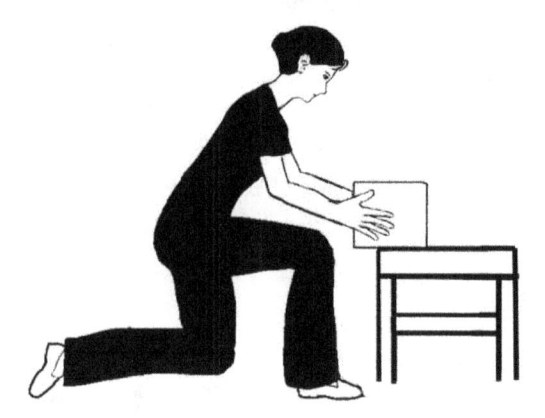

Another method which can be used to pick items up off the floor is called the golfer's reach. This movement is sometimes used by golfers to pick up the ball. Make sure you hold onto something sturdy to avoid losing your balance. Tip the upper body forward as you lift the back leg. This keeps your back straight versus bending at the waist as illustrated in the "incorrect" picture on page 37.

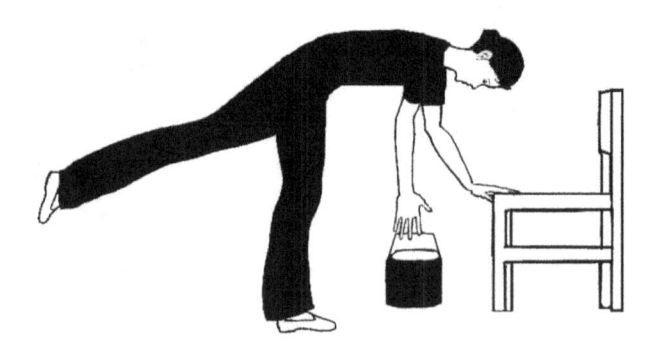

It is also important to think about how you reach items that are higher up. If an item is above shoulder height it is best to use a sturdy step stool.

**Incorrect**

Overreaching from shoulder, not a sturdy stance. Increased risk for falling backwards or dropping the item.

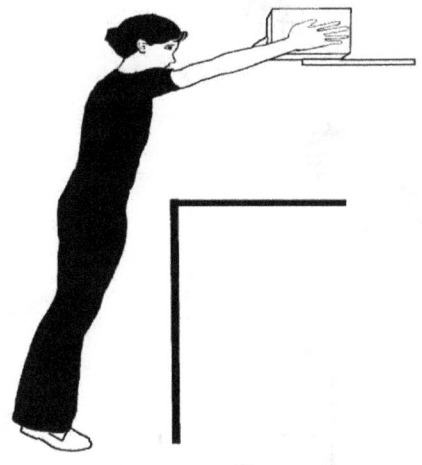

**Correct**

Place the item on a counter before stepping up onto or off of the stool. *Avoid* climbing up or stepping down from a stool with items in your hands! Keep the item close to you and get as close as you can to the shelf.

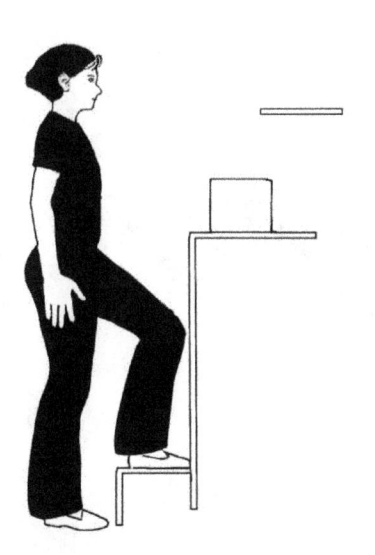

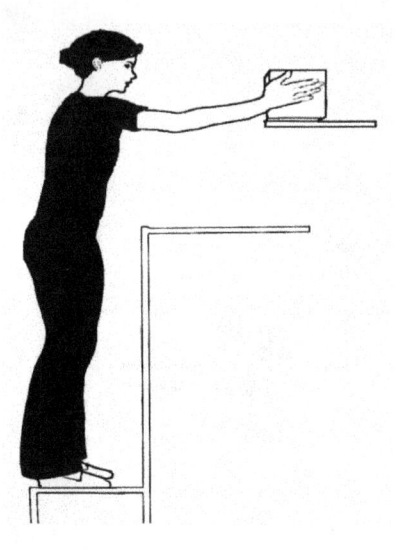

# Getting Down on the Floor

If you practice getting up and down from the floor on a regular basis, you will be more likely to be able to get up without help should you fall. People who fall at home must sometimes wait hours or even days before help arrives. When first attempting this, make sure you have someone around to help you until you can easily get up alone.

1. First make sure there is a sturdy chair nearby. Use the hip hinge motion (pg. 19) to place your hands on the chair.

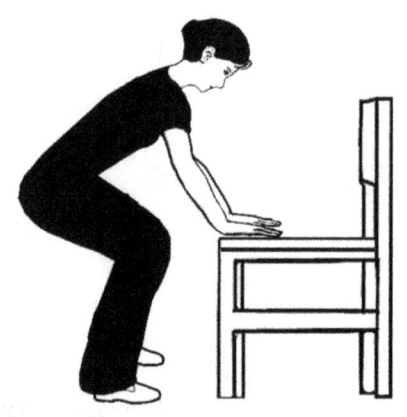

2. Then place one knee (whichever knee is more comfortable to do this with) on the floor. Continue to use the chair for support. Then come down on to all fours and move the chair away a bit.

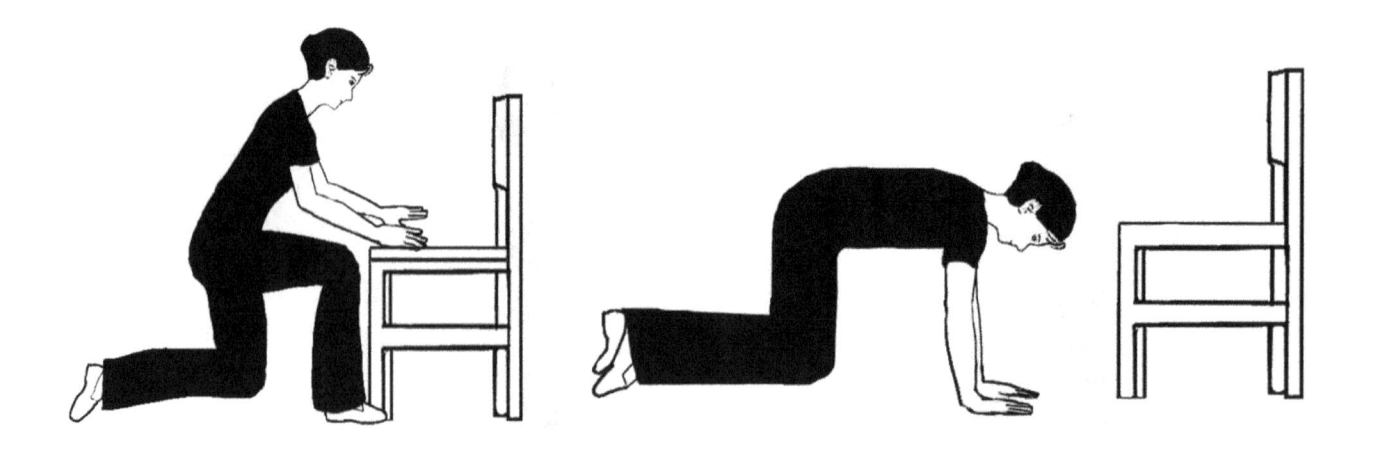

3. Then lower yourself down onto one hip, (whichever hip is more comfortable to bear weight on). Next, lower yourself down so that you are lying on your side.

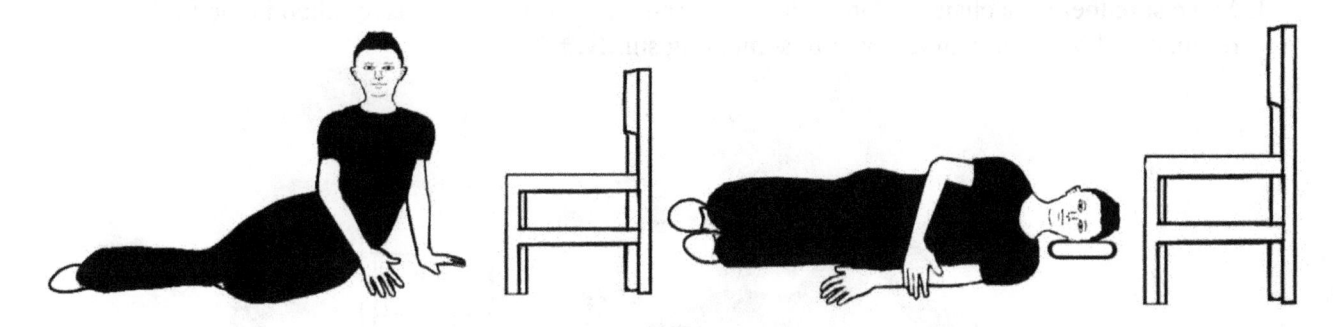

4. From here you can roll over onto your back.

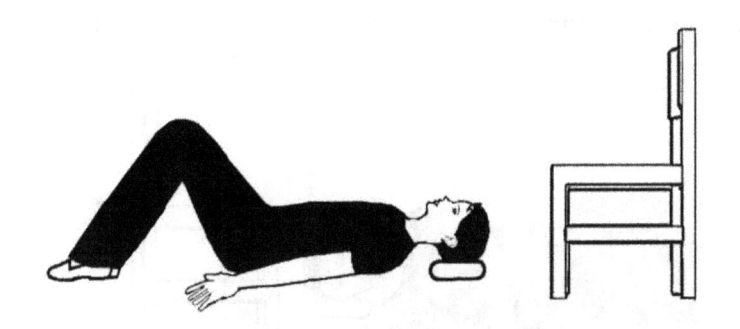

# Getting Up From the Floor

1. Make sure there is a chair or sturdy piece of furniture near by. If you have fallen in the middle of a room, crawl or scoot yourself over to something sturdy.

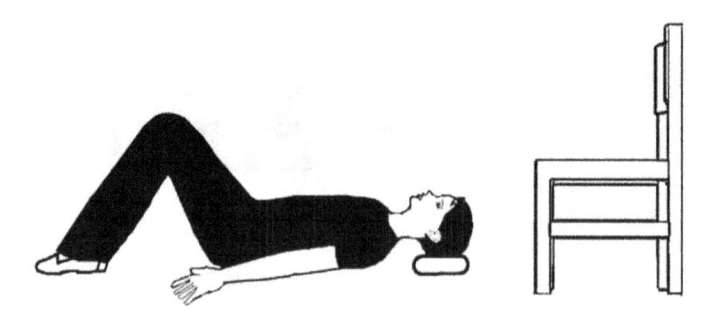

2. If you are on your back, first roll onto one side, (whichever side is more comfortable to bear weight on). Roll your body as a unit, the same as when getting out of bed.

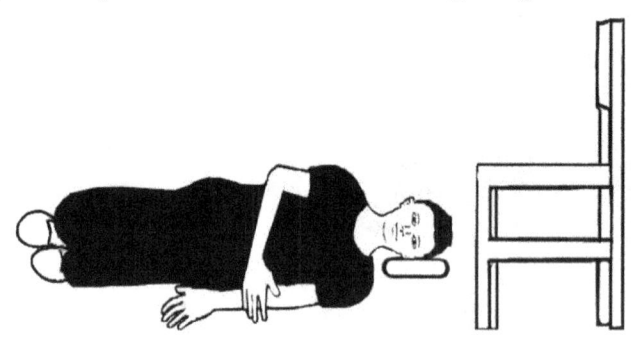

3. Then, using your arms, push up onto your hip.

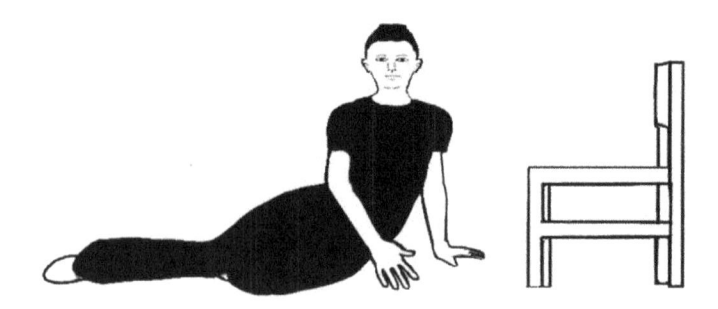

4. Next come up to all fours. Bring one foot forward so that you are on one knee (whichever knee is more comfortable to do this with). Place your hands on the chair for support.

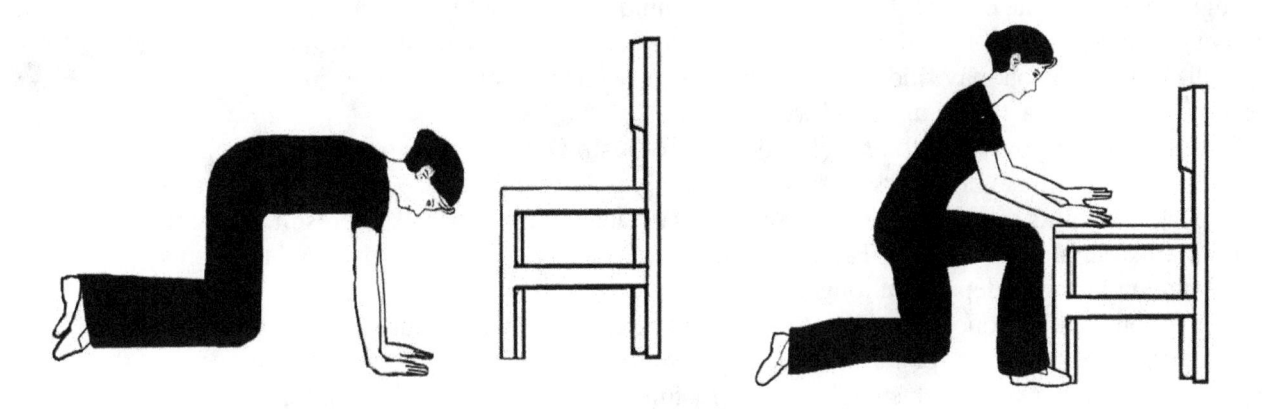

5. Using the chair for support, use the hip hinge motion to come up to standing. Remember to keep your back straight when transitioning from kneeling to standing.

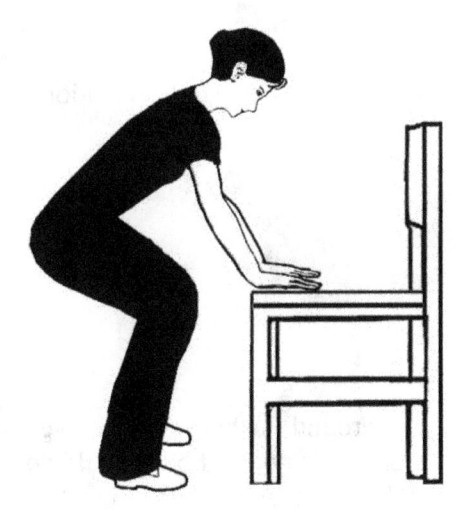

At least once per week practice getting up and down off the floor so you will be able to get yourself up if you fall.

## Summary

    Begin to incorporate correct body mechanics techniques on a daily basis. At first it may seem like daily tasks take longer, but with more practice using correct body mechanics will become more natural. With time you may find that you automatically correct yourself and eventually it will become common practice to use good working habits.

    To fully manage your symptoms and remain active, using correct body mechanics is an important step. Taking the time to do things correctly and safely will help to reduce the risk of falls and keep your back and joints safe from injury. Many falls and accidents happen as the result of rushing and not thinking our actions through. Taking the time to do things correctly helps avoid accidents enabling you to stay independent longer.

    Also if you have osteoporosis, you need to be diligent about your posture in order to avoid developing or worsening a forward rounded position or hunched back. Therefore using good body mechanics (keeping your back straight when brushing your teeth, putting on shoes, doing housework, etc). not only helps to avoid falls but also helps you keep the upper back muscles strong and the chest muscles stretched out. In contrast if you continually use poor body mechanics, you are training your body to develop a forward rounded posture.

    If you are experiencing significant difficulty with any of your daily activities, talk with your healthcare provider about attending physical or occupational therapy. Physical and occupational therapists are specially trained to work with you and your individual situation to help make everyday activities safer and more enjoyable.

> " I never fall. Then one day I was rushing around the house trying to get everything done. Next thing I knew I was on the floor. I was not hurt but I could not get back up and I could not reach the phone. Thankfully my daughter came by later that day and helped me up. It was a terrifying experience. In my osteoporosis class we started practicing the right way to get up and down. I am now doing exercises to improve my balance and being more careful. However, if I do fall again, I now know I can get up without help." - L.S. MA

# Chapter Two

## Diaphragmatic Breathing and Aerobic Exercise

*Identifying your enthusiasms requires courage and heroic creative vision.*
*You have to believe that what you want is possible for you.*
- Marsha Sinetar

One component of an exercise regimen is aerobic or cardiovascular exercise. This type of exercise includes any activity which is sustained and raises the heart and breathing rate. The purpose of aerobic exercise is to strengthen the heart and lungs, train the body to utilize oxygen more efficiently and help maintain a healthy weight and blood pressure.

Examples of aerobic activities include:
- Walking
- Biking
- Swimming
- Aerobic dancing

Regular aerobic exercise can help:
- Take off excess weight and maintain a healthy weight
- Strengthen the heart and lungs
- Improve stamina and endurance
- Reduce stress
- Improve mood and combat depression
- Help control high blood pressure and high cholesterol
- Aerobic exercise that is weight bearing helps to strengthen bones

### *How Often Should You Exercise*

Thirty to forty five minutes of aerobic exercise on most days of the week is recommended. If you have not been exercising regularly, this would be too much to start with. If you are just beginning to exercise either for the first time or after being away from it for a while, try for 5 to 10 minutes two to three times per week. Then, each week try to add one to two minutes until you can comfortably do 15 minutes three times per week. From there keep adding more and more time slowly and eventually add additional days. A common mistake made by many is to start off too vigorously. This leads to muscle soreness and fatigue; making it difficult to keep exercising. Starting slowly and increasing gradually; allows the body to adapt to the exercise. While one can expect to feel some stiffness at the start, your routine should not cause pain or discomfort to the point where it restricts you from doing daily activities.

## *How Hard Should You Exercise*

Before beginning aerobic exercise, make sure you warm-up by taking a short walk or performing the "rhythmic limbering" exercises included in this chapter. The goal of aerobic exercise is to raise the heart and breathing rate to a point where you will benefit from the routine. During aerobic classes it is commonly recommended to take your pulse (or your heart rate) during the exercise session, with a goal of sustaining it at a level equal to 60 to 80 percent of your heart's maximum ability. However, many medications can interfere with your heart rate. For example some heart medications work to keep your heart rate lower. When you start exercising the medication will continue to try to lower your heart rate. This means you may be working very hard but your medication is working to keep lowering your heart rate. If you continue to try to increase your heart rate to 60 to 80 percent, you may be putting yourself at risk for injury. In other words, taking your heart rate may not be providing you with an accurate picture of how hard you are actually working.

Another concern with taking your heart rate is that many people have a hard time locating their pulse. This can often cause people to stop exercising while they try to find their pulse. When you stop the heart rate drops which interferes with keeping the exercise at a steady pace. Given this, many people choose to use a scale known as the Rating of Perceived Exertion. This scale assigns a number to describe how hard you feel you are working. It is a self-rating technique you can do periodically during your routine to judge if you are working at the right level to gain benefits. At periods throughout your routine take a moment to use the following scale to rate how you are doing.

The Rating of Perceived Exertion scale is as follows:

1 No effort, resting
2 Very, Very Light
3 Very Light
4 Fairly Light
5 Moderate
6 Somewhat Hard
7 Hard
8 Very Hard
9 Very, Very Hard
10 Maximum Effort

For your aerobic program, you should gradually work up to a level between 5 to 7. Working at a level of 1 to 4 will not be vigorous enough to get the full benefit from your routine. Working above level 7 may lead to soreness, injury and fatigue.

Another way to test how hard you are working is the talk test. While exercising you should not be so out of breath that you can not even answer a yes or no question. If you are gasping for breath just to say a few words you are working too hard. If on the other hand you are able to carry on a full conversation with no trouble, you may not be exercising hard enough.

Using music for the aerobic component helps to ensure that you are working at a good pace in order to raise your heart rate high enough to get benefits. It also can make the time go by faster. Using music is also a good way to time your routine. However long you are aiming to exercise - five minutes, ten minutes or a longer, try making a tape or CD that plays the same amount of time you want your routine to be. In the classes we teach, our music is approximately 120 beats per minute. To determine the beats per minute of a song do the following:

- Get a stopwatch or watch with a second hand
- Play the music you wish to use
- Tap to the beat of the song with your hand or foot
- Count how many times you tap in a 15-second period
- You should count about 30 beats.

If you find that this speed of music too fast to keep up with, start with slower music and gradually work up to music that is 120 beats per minute.

The following movements are the ones we teach in our program. They move the body in a variety of directions to fully work the joints and muscles. Challenging the body to travel in different directions such as forward, backwards, and sideways helps to improve balance. Because there are many other ways to move the body, you may wish to vary this routine with other movements you know. Aerobic exercise can be done standing, standing and holding onto a chair or counter for support, or while seated. *Try to do as much as you can standing.* This will help to improve balance and provide weight bearing exercise to help strengthen the bones, as well as improving your cardiovascular health.

Experiment with the different variations to find the right option for you. You can do some of each. For example, if you are new to exercise or having a day when you are not feeling well, you may choose to do a few repetitions standing and then a few repetitions seated. As with everything in this program explore different approaches to see what feels best. The movements will be shown one per page with instructions. The last page will list all the movements together and provides sample sequences so you can move through your routine more smoothly.

It is important to let the body cool down slowly after exercise. After completing aerobic activity, continue with some type of gentle movement for another three to five minutes to let the heart and breathing rate slowly adjust back to their pre-exercise level.

# Exploring the Cardiovascular and Circulatory System.
## *Why I need to exercise my heart*

The cardiovascular system is made up of the heart, blood, and blood vessels. The circulatory system is your body's delivery system. Blood leaving the heart delivers oxygen and nutrients to every part of the body. On the way back to the heart, the blood picks up and carries away waste products.

### *The heart*

The heart is a very important muscle of the body. In an average lifetime the heart beats more than two and a half billion times and pumps nearly 4000 gallons of blood each day. It pumps blood around your body supplying the cells with nutrients and removing waste. It contracts on average between 60 to 80 times a minute, more if you are exercising or exerting yourself. This number is known as your "heart rate."

The heart contains four chambers, and is shaped and sized roughly like a man's fist. The top two chambers are called the atria and the bottom two chambers are called the ventricles.

Aorta - Carries oxygenated blood to the body.

Superior Vena Cava

Right Atrium – Receives blood from the body

Right Ventricle – Pumps blood to the lungs to be oxygenated

Inferior Vena Cava

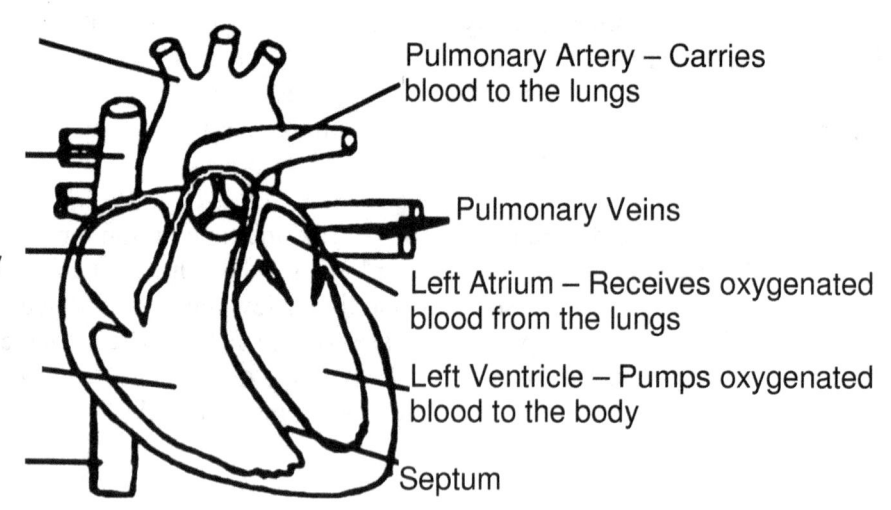

Pulmonary Artery – Carries blood to the lungs

Pulmonary Veins

Left Atrium – Receives oxygenated blood from the lungs

Left Ventricle – Pumps oxygenated blood to the body

Septum

**Blood Pressure**

Blood pressure measures the pressure the blood exerts against the walls of the arteries and it changes constantly according to the body's needs. The systolic or top number represents when the heart pumps and the blood ventricles contract. The diastolic or bottom number represents the heart at rest when the ventricles relax. When blood pressure is measured it is recorded as a fraction such as 120/80 mmHg.

**Exercise and your heart**

Regular aerobic exercise is the best method of keeping the heart muscle strong and healthy as it places specific demands on the body. During aerobic exercise the muscles demand more oxygen-rich blood and give off more carbon dioxide and other waste. To accomplish this the heart must beat faster and pump more blood with each beat to meet these demands. This means that your heart rate and blood pressure must increase in order to supply the working muscles with an increased need for blood and oxygen.

The effects of regular exercise will depend on the type, duration, frequency and intensity of training. Since the heart muscle must work harder to accommodate the increased needs during exercise, the heart muscle will become stronger and more efficient. When you give your heart this kind of workout on a regular basis your heart will become better at its main job, delivering blood and oxygen to all parts of your body. When you follow a program of regular aerobic exercise, over time your heart grows stronger and can meet the muscles' demands without as much effort.

Regular aerobic exercise can:
- Increase the size of major coronary vessels, making it easier for the blood to flow to all regions of the heart - in other words there is more space and less resistance for the blood to flow through as it travels throughout the body
- Increase the size and pumping ability of the heart. As with all of the muscles in the body, when the heart muscle is stressed through exercise it gets stronger
- Increase the number of capillaries in the body thereby aiding in the distribution of blood
- Lower blood pressure due to a stronger more efficient system
- Lead to a decrease in body fat and weight so there is less area for the body to have to supply blood to
- Lower resting heart rate, meaning that the heart will not have to work as hard at rest

Regular aerobic exercise produces a more efficient system that recovers quicker. This means that when you stop the aerobic exercise session your blood pressure, rate of breathing and heart rate will recover and return to their pre-exercise levels more quickly then they could before you started an exercise program. This means that your body is adapting to the exercise program and is becoming more efficient.

# Exploring the Respiratory System
## *Why I need to exercise my lungs*

You breathe with the help of your diaphragm and other muscles in your chest and abdomen. These muscles literally change the space and pressure inside the body to accommodate breathing. Your lungs are like a pair of balloons that expand when you inhale. When you inhale, your diaphragm drops down so the lung cavity can expand and take in air. When you exhale the muscles squeeze your rib cage, your diaphragm moves upwards, your lungs begin to collapse, and the air is pushed up and out of your body.

### *How the oxygen you breathe gets into the blood*

You breathe in about 20 times per minute. Every minute you inhale approximately 13 pints of air. In the course of a day, approximately 8,000 to 9,000 liters of inhaled air meets 8,000 to 10,000 liters of blood pumped in by the heart through the pulmonary artery.

The air you inhale passes through the nasal passages that filter, heat, and moisten the air before it flows into the back of the throat. The air then flows down through the trachea (windpipe) to where the lower ribs meet the center of your chest. Here your windpipe divides into two tubes, which lead to the lungs. Inside each of your lungs tubes called bronchi branch into still even smaller tubes much like the branches of a tree. At the end of these tubes are millions of tiny sacs called alveoli. Here, the red blood cells interact with these sacs to trade in the old carbon dioxide that your body's cells have made, for some new oxygen you have just breathed in.

The "new" oxygen passes through the walls of each alveoli into the tiny capillaries that surround them and enters the blood, where it is carried by red blood cells to the heart. The heart then sends the oxygen-rich blood through arteries and capillaries to all the cells in the body.

Veins then carry the oxygen-depleted blood back to the heart and then onto the lungs. Here, the carbon dioxide and waste picked up by the alveoli travels through the lungs, back up your windpipe and it is expelled with every exhale.

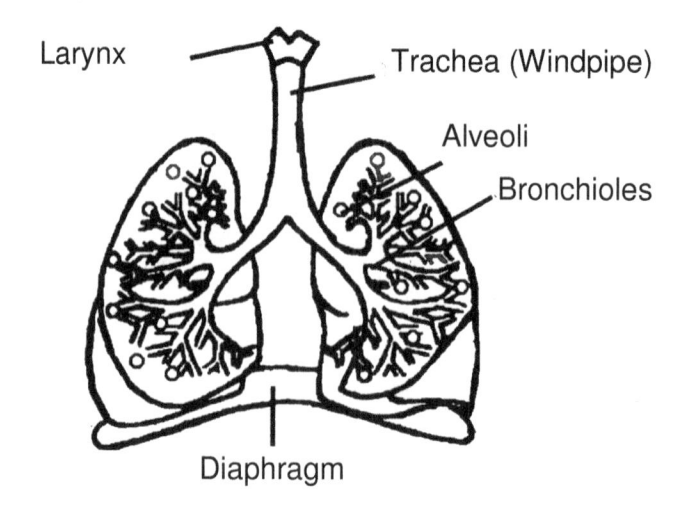

*Exercise and your respiratory system*

During exercise the muscles use more oxygen than when they are at rest. At rest the muscles take up 6 ml per 100 ml of oxygen. During heavy exercise the muscles can take up as much as 17 ml per 100 ml. Aerobic exercise places demands on the system which results in a stronger respiratory system, making it more efficient at delivering and processing oxygen in the body.

Cardiorespiratory endurance (the health of our heart and lungs) refers to the body's ability to sustain prolonged activity. The endurance of this system can be tested by measuring the highest rate of oxygen consumption attainable during maximal exertion. This level of maximal exertion is known as your "V02 max." When you reach this level your body can no longer deliver oxygen as quickly as your muscles need to receive it. Thus you will not be able to continue the activity you were doing for much longer. Regular aerobic activity has been shown to increase this level, allowing you to perform activities for longer periods at a higher intensity.

Regular aerobic exercise brings about changes in the body's cardiorespiratory system enabling it to function more effectively. Much like the heart during exercise, aerobic exercise forces the lungs to work harder and faster to deliver the needed oxygen, which strengthens and conditions them. Exercise is good for every part of your body, especially your lungs and heart. When you take part in regular exercise your lungs require more air to give your cells the extra oxygen they need. As you breathe more deeply and take in more air, your lungs become stronger and more efficient at supplying your body with the air it needs for exercise and everyday activities.

Below are some of the benefits of regular aerobic exercise.

- Makes your heart and cardiorespiratory system stronger and more efficient
- Improves lung capacity. This is very beneficial for those with osteoporosis. An increase in lung capacity means that you do not get out of breath as quickly during all types of activity such as climbing stairs and walking uphill
- Strengthens the diaphragm muscle.
- Decreases fatigue. After approximately four to eight weeks of participating in regular aerobic exercise you may notice that you feel less tired during exercise and everyday activities.
- Induces sleep. Many of our class participants who do regular aerobic exercise notice that they sleep better at night.
- Increases your tolerance for exercise. You will find you can exercise longer and at a harder pace then when you started.

# Diaphragmatic Breathing

Before beginning to explore different movement techniques it is important to discuss breathing. Most people take shallow breaths moving only the chest and shoulders. When taking shallow breaths the diaphragm is not used to its full capacity. Also, having osteoporosis can cause a decrease in lung capacity as the back and shoulders round forward and there is less room for the lungs to move. It is more efficient and beneficial to learn to breathe more deeply, using the diaphragm and moving the abdominal cavity. Learning to breathe abdominally (from the diaphragm) also helps to promote relaxation, which improves physical and mental health. This occurs since belly breathing is a more efficient way for the body to take in oxygen and remove carbon dioxide with the least effort.

The diaphragm is a large, dome-shaped muscle that contracts rhythmically and continually, and most of the time involuntarily. The diaphragm sits beneath the lungs and above the abdominal cavity. When you exhale the abdominal muscles should contract, allowing the diaphragm to move upward, so the air is fully expelled from the lungs. During inhalation the abdominal muscles should relax and move outwards, allowing the diaphragm muscle to move downward, so the lungs can fully expand.

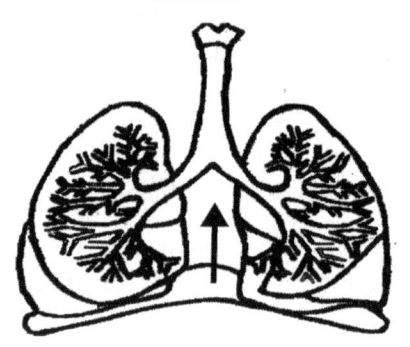

**Exhale:**

Diaphragm moves up

**Inhale:**

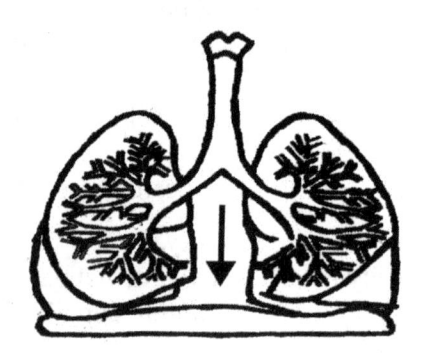

Diaphragm moves down

Though breathing is an automatic function, the movements of the diaphragm can be controlled voluntarily with training. Benefits of diaphragmatic breathing include:

- A more efficient exchange of oxygen and carbon dioxide
- Promotion of general relaxation
- Improved circulation
- Removal of waste products from the blood
- Slower heart rate and breathing rate
- Calming of the mind

This method of breathing may feel awkward because we were often taught to pull in the stomach muscles as we inhale, but this actually restricts the movement of the diaphragm. However, with practice this deeper form of breathing will become more natural. The easiest way to practice diaphragmatic breathing is lying down, the second easiest is while standing, and most difficult is while seated. You can begin to try this deep breathing by lying on your bed or couch. Then try it while standing, and then seated. We will use this breath during every exercise and movement in this book. This breathing technique should be done as much as possible through the nose rather than the mouth. Breathing through the nose is more efficient and relaxing for the body because the nasal cavity is better designed to purify and warm the air. If you are experiencing any type of respiratory or sinus concerns, or if you become dizzy while breathing strictly through the nose, try inhaling only through the nose and then exhaling through pursed lips.

## Belly Breathing Lying Down

Lie on your back with a pillow under your head if needed.
Place one hand on your belly and the other on your chest.
As you exhale through the nose gently contract the abdominal muscles and push all of the air out of your belly and lungs. The hand on the belly should move down. Think of moving the belly towards the floor.

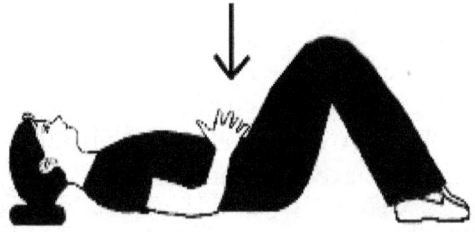

As you inhale through the nose let the abdominal muscles relax and let the belly rise first. With the inhalation the hand on the belly should move up and the hand on the chest should stay still. Think of moving the belly towards the ceiling. Then let the chest and the hand on the chest rise. It may take some practice to have the belly move first, or at all.

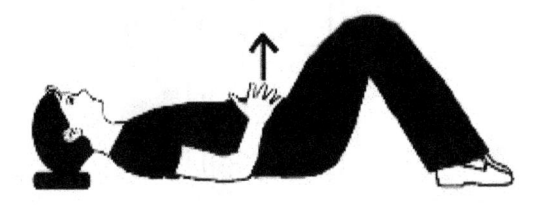

## Belly Breathing Seated

Use the correct sitting posture. Sit at the front edge of the chair and away from the back of the chair. Feet should be flat on the floor The shoulders stay down and relaxed.

Place one hand on your belly and the other on your chest. As you exhale through the nose, gently contract your abdominal muscles and push all of the air out of your belly and lungs. The hand on your belly should move inwards. Think of moving your belly towards the back of the chair.

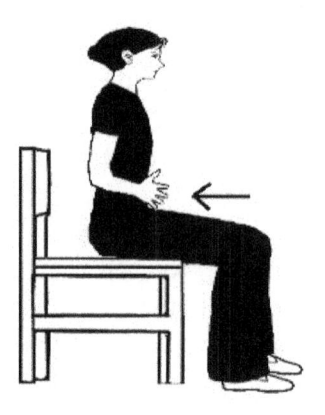

As you inhale through the nose let the belly rise first. Your belly and the hand on your belly should move outwards with the inhalation. Then let the chest and the hand on the chest rise next. It may take some practice to have the belly move first, or at all. Do not let the shoulders rise up when inhaling. They should stay down and relaxed the entire time.

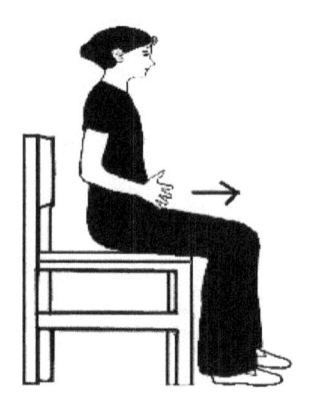

# Rhythmic Limbering Exercises

Before beginning any exercise routine it is important to "warm-up" the body. "Warming-up" simply means preparing the joints and muscles for movement, and allowing the heart and breathing rate to increase slowly. If we do not take the time to warm up the body correctly we risk injury to the joints and muscles. The following exercises help loosen the joints and muscles and bring oxygen to the body, which can make the body more receptive to aerobic, strength training, and flexibility exercises. The following are some basic movements you can do to help prepare the body for aerobic exercise. The following exercises are shown both seated and standing and you ant to try to do as much as you can standing.

## Breathe and Reach

Before starting check your posture. Stand or sit up straight, bring the hips under the shoulders, and think about pushing the crown of the head up to the ceiling without lifting the chin. Arms are down by your sides. Inhale bringing the arms up overhead. Make sure the shoulders stay down. As you exhale lower the arms back to your sides. Repeat 3 times.

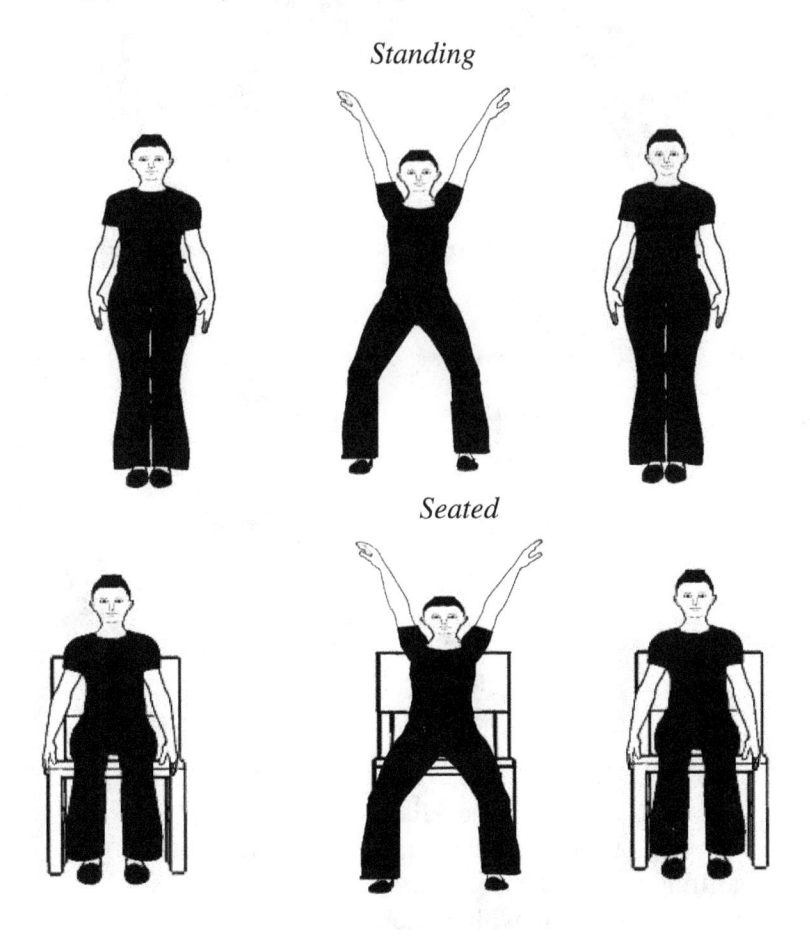

*Standing*

*Seated*

## Squat and Reach Overhead

Before starting check your posture. Stand or sit up straight, bring the hips under the shoulders, and think about pushing the crown of the head up to the ceiling without lifting the chin.

Squat down only as far as you can without hurting your knees. Then stand up and reach the right arm overhead. Squat down again. Then stand up and reach the left arm overhead. Do 8-12 repetitions alternating right to left.

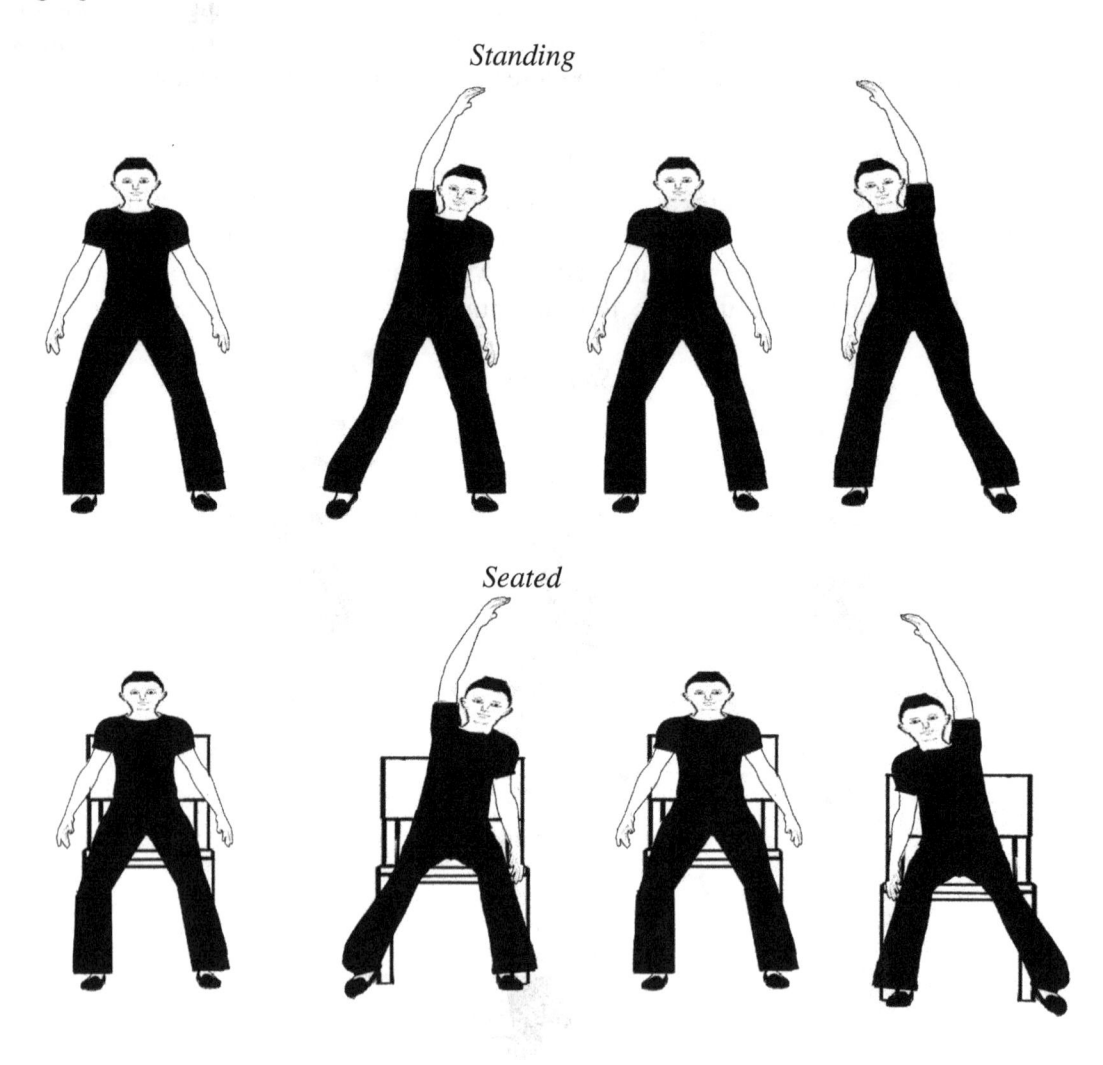

*Standing*

*Seated*

Checklist
- ✓ Stand or sit up straight. Think of pushing the crown of the head up to the ceiling without lifting the chin
- ✓ Do as much as you can standing without holding on
- ✓ Only squat as low as your knees comfortably allow
- ✓ Breathe

## Squat and Reach Forward

Before starting check your posture. Stand or sit up straight, bring the hips under the shoulders, and think about pushing the crown of the head up to the ceiling without lifting the chin.

Squat down only as far as you can without hurting your knees. Then stand up and reach the right arm across the body chest height. Be careful to not twist the back or knees, keep the hips and shoulders facing forward. Squat down again. Then stand up and reach the left arm across the body chest height. Do 8-12 repetitions alternating right to left.

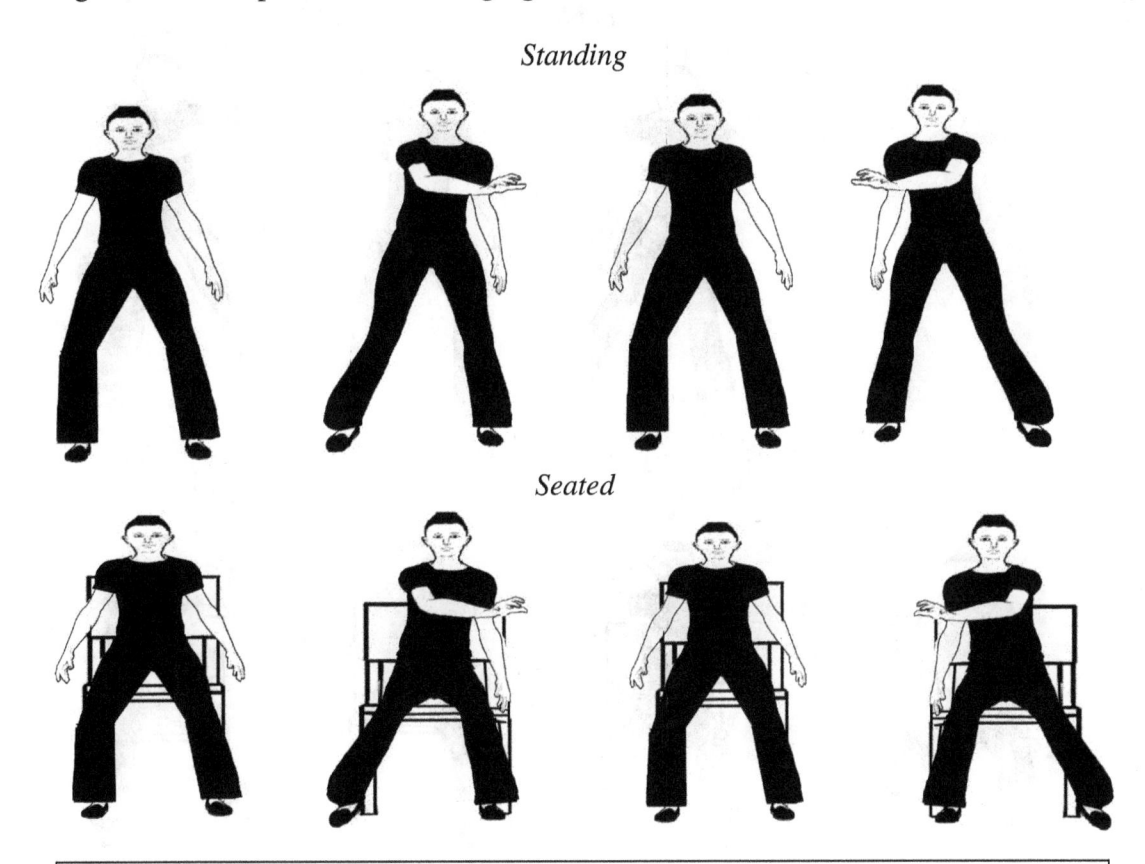

*Standing*

*Seated*

Checklist
- ✓ Stand or sit up straight. Think of pushing the crown of the head up to the ceiling without lifting the chin
- ✓ Do as much as you can standing without holding on
- ✓ Only squat as low as your knees comfortably allow
- ✓ Keep the hips and shoulders facing forward
- ✓ Do not twist the knees or back
- ✓ Breathe

## Squat and Swing The Arms

Before starting check your posture. Stand or sit up straight, bring the hips under the shoulders, and think about pushing the crown of the head up to the ceiling without lifting the chin.

Squat down only as far as you can without hurting your knees. Then stand up and swing both arms across the body to the right. Be careful to not twist the back or knees. Squat down again. Then stand up and swing both arms across the body to the left. Do 8-12 repetitions alternating right to left.

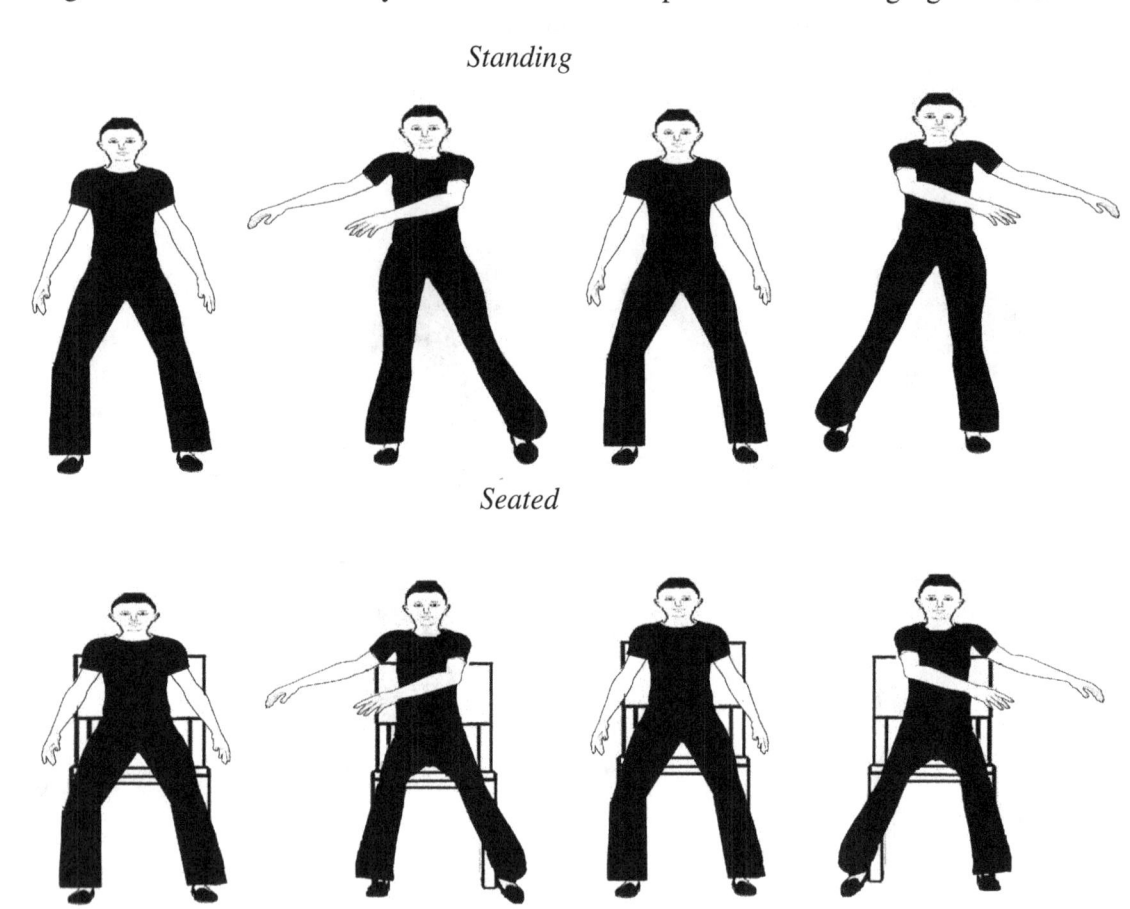

*Standing*

*Seated*

Checklist
- ✓ Stand or sit up straight. Think of pushing the crown of the head up to the ceiling without lifting the chin
- ✓ Do as much as you can standing without holding on
- ✓ Only squat as low as your knees comfortably allow
- ✓ Do not twist the back or the knees
- ✓ Breathe

## Heel To Toe Rock

Before starting check your posture. Stand or sit up straight, bring the hips under the shoulders, and think about pushing the crown of the head up to the ceiling without lifting the chin.

Rock forward tapping the back toe on the floor and lift the arms up to the front. Then rock back tapping the front heel and swing the arms back. Continue back and forth 8-12 times.

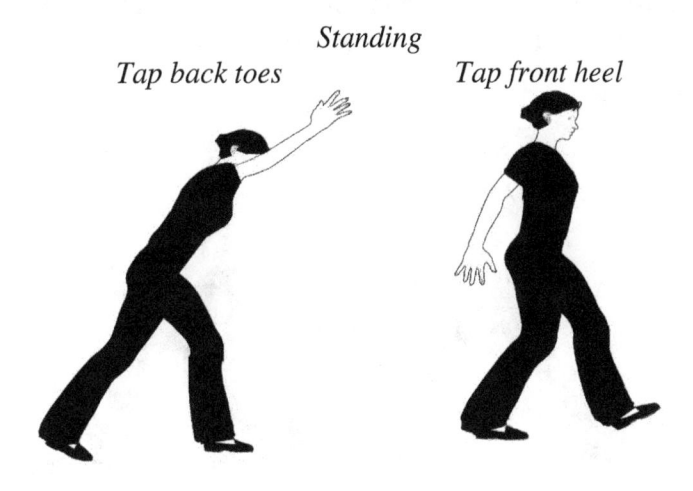

*Standing*
*Tap back toes*    *Tap front heel*

*Seated*
Lift the heels off the floor.

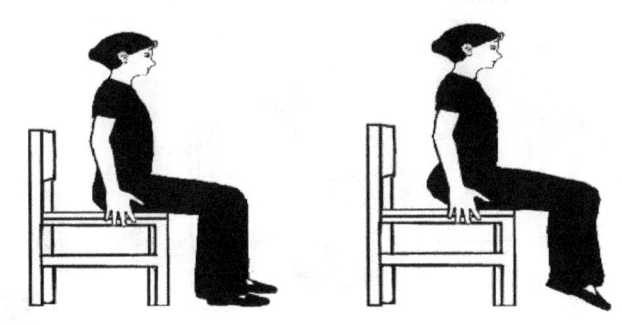

### Checklist
- ✓ Stand or sit up straight. Think of pushing the crown of the head up to the ceiling without lifting the chin
- ✓ Do as much as you can standing without holding on
- ✓ Do not twist the back or the knees
- ✓ Breathe

# Knee Drop

Before starting check your posture. Stand or sit up straight, bring the hips under the shoulders, and think about pushing the crown of the head up to the ceiling without lifting the chin.

Stand in a lunge position with the right foot forward and the left foot back. Support yourself with your hands on your thighs. Line the front knee over the front ankle and make sure the front knee does not go past the front ankle. Drop the back knee towards the floor. Only go as low as your knees will allow. Come back up. Repeat 8-12 times and then switch to the other side. You can hold onto a chair or counter if needed to maintain balance and then try to work up to not holding on.

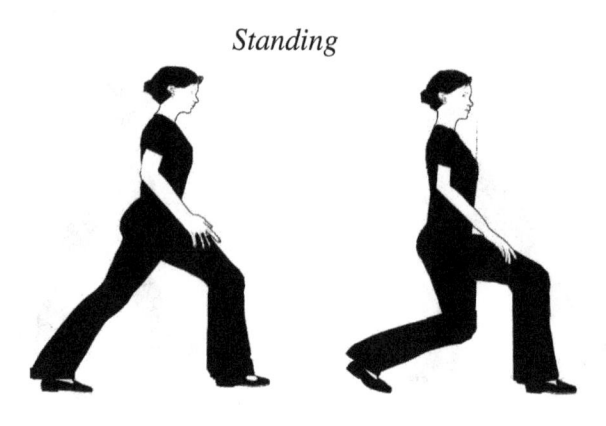

*Standing*

*Seated*
Alternately pull the heels under the chair.

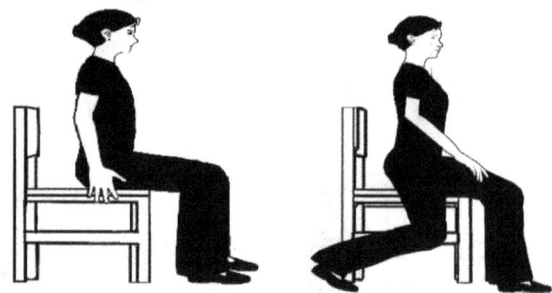

| Checklist |
| --- |
| ✓ Stand or sit up straight. Think of pushing the crown of the head up to the ceiling without lifting the chin |
| ✓ Do as much as you can standing without holding on |
| ✓ Only squat as low as your knees comfortably allow |
| ✓ Keep the front knee aligned over the front ankle |
| ✓ Breathe |

## Hamstring Stretch

Before starting check your posture. Stand or sit up straight, bring the hips under the shoulders, and think about pushing the crown of the head up to the ceiling without lifting the chin.

Stand in a lunge position with the right leg forward and the left leg back. Make sure both the front toes and the back toes are pointing forward and do not turn the back leg out. Bend your front knee and press your back heel to the floor. Line the front knee over the front ankle and make sure the front knee does not go past the front ankle. You should be able to look down at your right knee and see your toes.

Hold for 5-10 deep breaths. Repeat on the other side. You can hold onto a chair or counter if needed to maintain balance and then try to work up to not holding on.

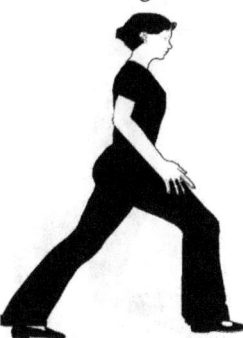

*Standing*

*Seated*

When seated make sure you keep the back straight. Come forward with your chest and do not round the back.

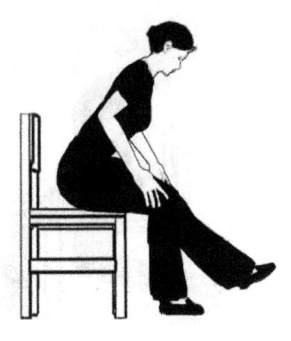

---

Checklist
- ✓ Stand or sit up straight. Think of pushing the crown of the head up to the ceiling without lifting the chin
- ✓ Do as much as you can standing without holding on
- ✓ When standing keep the front knee aligned over the front ankle
- ✓ Breathe

## Quadriceps Stretch

Before starting check your posture. Stand or sit up straight, bring the hips under the shoulders, and think about pushing the crown of the head up to the ceiling without lifting the chin.

Stand in a lunge position with the right leg forward and the left leg back. Make sure both the front toes and the back toes are pointing forward and do not turn the back leg out. Drop your back knee down as far as you comfortably can. Line the front knee over the front ankle and make sure the front knee does not go past the front ankle. You should be able to look down at your right knee and see your toes.

Hold for 5-10 deep breaths. Repeat on the other side. You can hold onto a chair or counter if needed to maintain balance and then try to work up to not holding on.

*Standing*

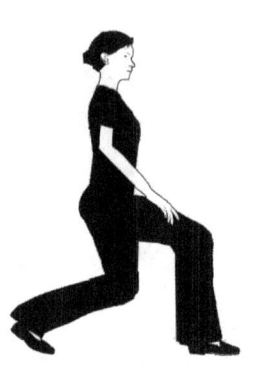

*Seated*

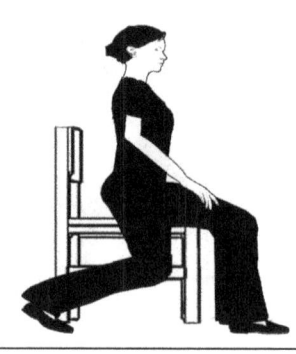

| Checklist |
|---|
| ✓ Stand or sit up straight. Think of pushing the crown of the head up to the ceiling without lifting the chin |
| ✓ Do as much as you can standing without holding on |
| ✓ Only squat as low as your knees comfortably allow |
| ✓ Keep the front knee aligned over the front ankle |
| ✓ Breathe |

## Shin Stretch

Before starting check your posture. Stand or sit up straight, bring the hips under the shoulders, and think about pushing the crown of the head up to the ceiling without lifting the chin.

Bring the right heel forward. Lean slightly forward – leaning from the hips. Do not round the back or shoulders, keep your back straight. Drop the toes to the floor and then lift the toes up. Repeat 8-12 times.

After completing 8-12 repetitions hold the toes up for a stretch. Hold for 5-10 deep breaths. Repeat other side. You can hold onto a chair or counter if needed to maintain balance and then try to work up to not holding on.

*Standing lifting toes*

*Standing Stretch*

*Seated lifting toes*

*Seated stretch*

Checklist
- ✓ Stand or sit up straight. Think of pushing the crown of the head up to the ceiling without lifting the chin
- ✓ Do as much as you can standing without holding on
- ✓ When standing lean forward from the hips. Do not round the back
- ✓ Breathe

# Aerobic Exercises

## Marching In Place
Alternately lift the feet off the floor and swing the arms.

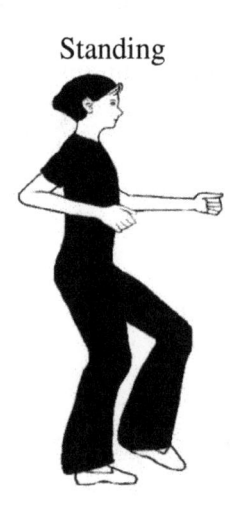

Standing

Standing with assistance
Do not lean on the chair or grab it too tightly. Let your legs work to support you.

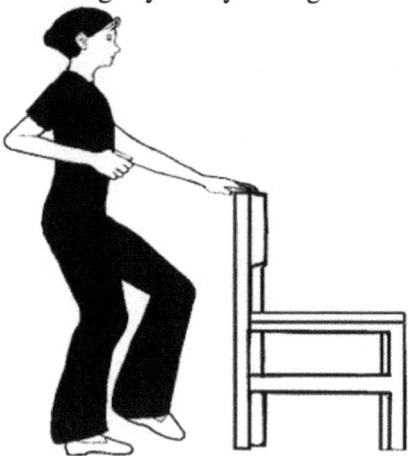

*Seated*

You can also march in place while sitting in a chair. Sit up straight and away from the back of the chair as much as possible.

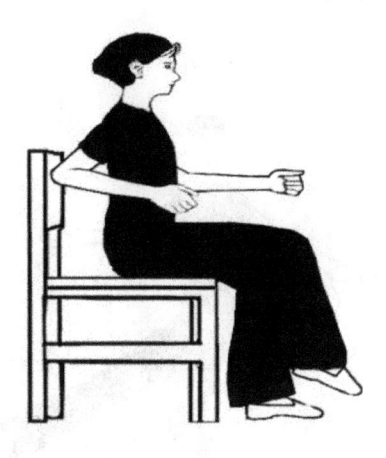

---

### Checklist
- ✓ Stand or sit up straight. Think of pushing the crown of the head up to the ceiling without lifting the chin
- ✓ Do as much as you can standing without holding on
- ✓ Swing your arms, using opposite arm to leg
- ✓ Try to avoid swinging the same arm as leg, which can bring you out of balance
- ✓ Focus on picking the feet up so that they come completely off the floor
- ✓ Periodically use the Rating of Perceived Exertion or talk test (pg. 46) to check if you are exercising at the right level
- ✓ Breathe

## Alternate Straight Leg Kicks

Alternately kick forward with a straight leg. Kick as high as you can keeping your balance and your back straight. Swing the opposite arm to leg.

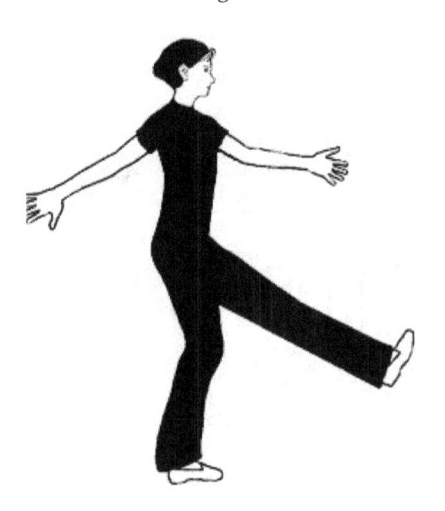

*Standing*

Standing with assistance
Do not lean on the chair or grab it too tight. Let your legs work to support you.

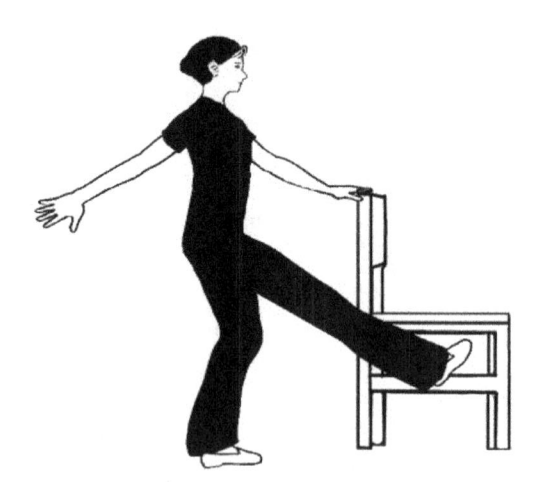

## Seated

You can also kick in place while sitting in a chair. Sit up straight and away from the back of the chair as much as possible.

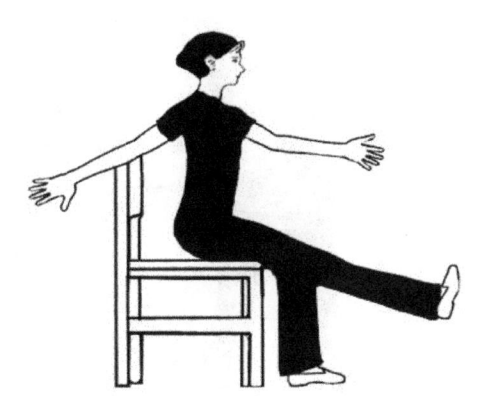

---

### Checklist
- ✓ Stand or sit up straight. Think of pushing the crown of the head up to the ceiling without lifting the chin
- ✓ Do as much as you can standing without holding on
- ✓ Swing your arms, using opposite arm to leg
- ✓ Try to avoid swinging the same arm as leg, which can bring you out of balance
- ✓ Focus on keeping the knee straight
- ✓ Periodically use the Rating of Perceived Exertion or talk test (pg. 46) to check if you are exercising at the right level
- ✓ Breathe

## Stepping Side to Side

Standing

Stand with feet together.   Step out to the right.   Bring the left foot to the right foot

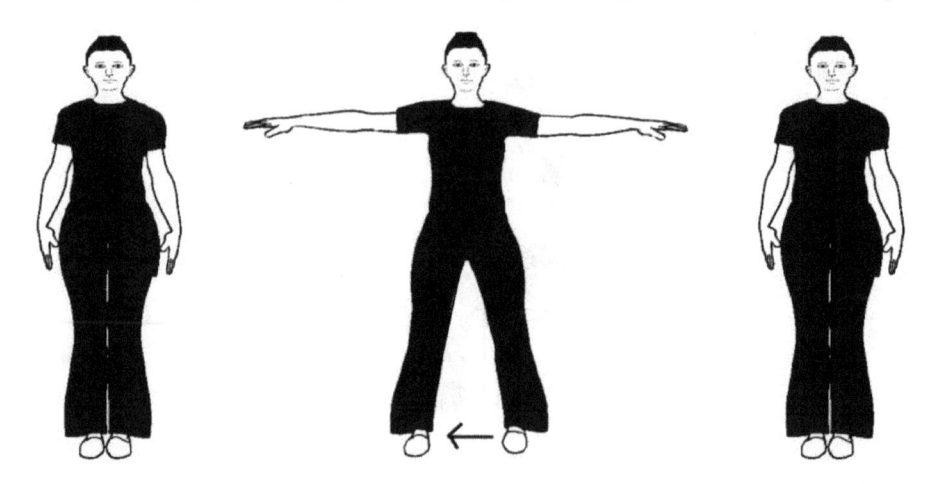

Stand with feet together.   Step out to the left.   Bring the right foot to the left foot

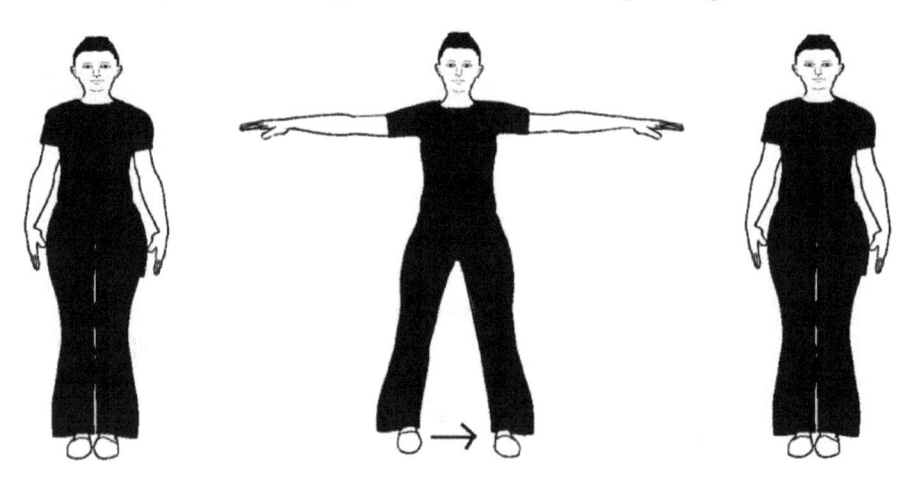

Continue stepping from right to left. Try to swing the arms up to shoulder height.

## Standing with Assistance

Do not lean on the chair or counter or grab it too tightly. Let your legs work to support you.
Step out to the left and bring the right foot to the left.

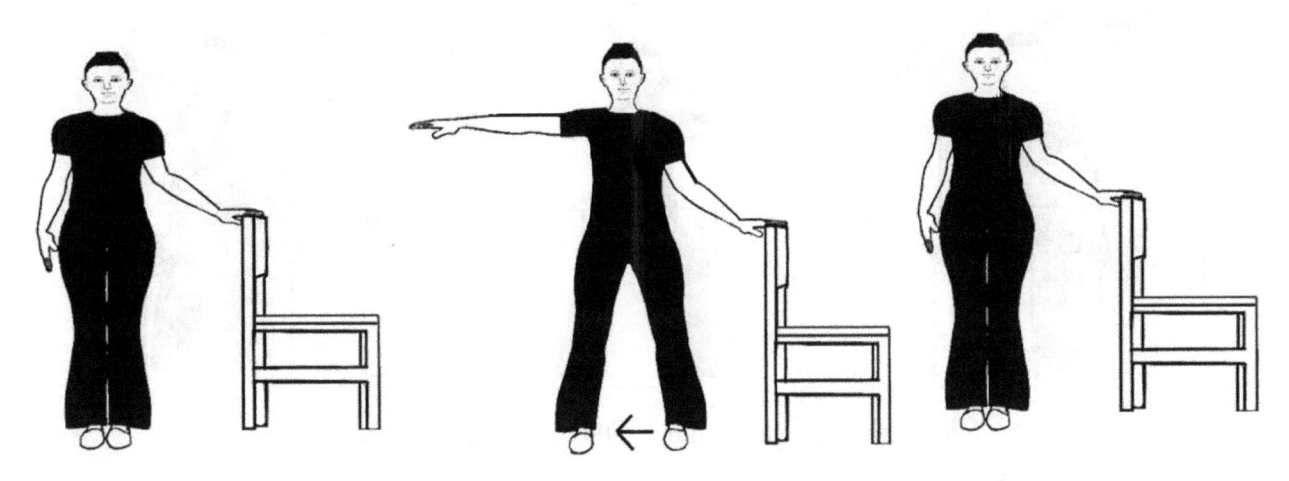

Continue stepping from right to left. Try to swing the arm up to shoulder height.

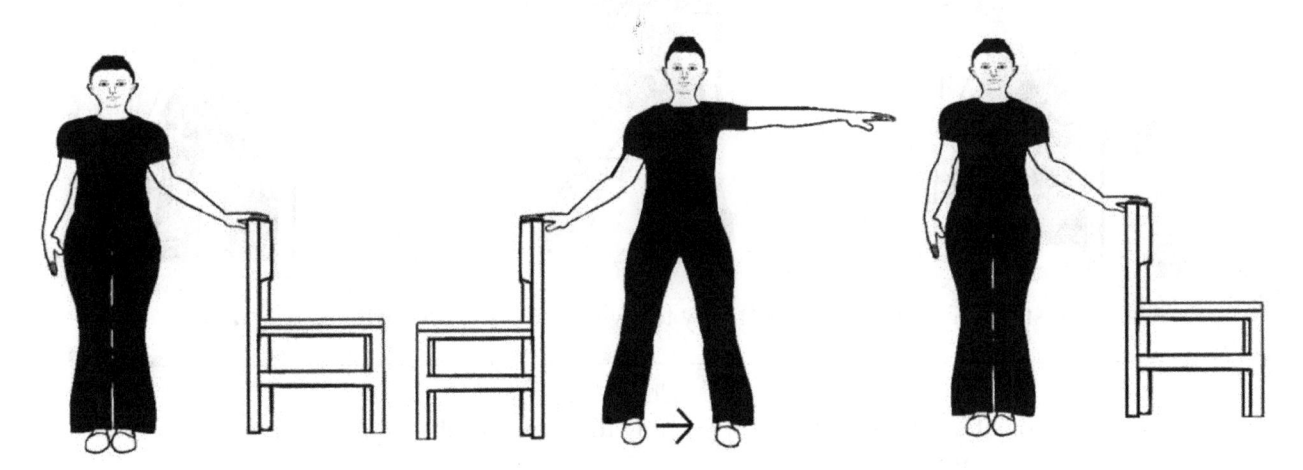

## Seated

You can also step side to side while sitting in a chair. Sit up straight and away from the back of the chair as much as possible. Step out to the right and bring the left foot to the right.

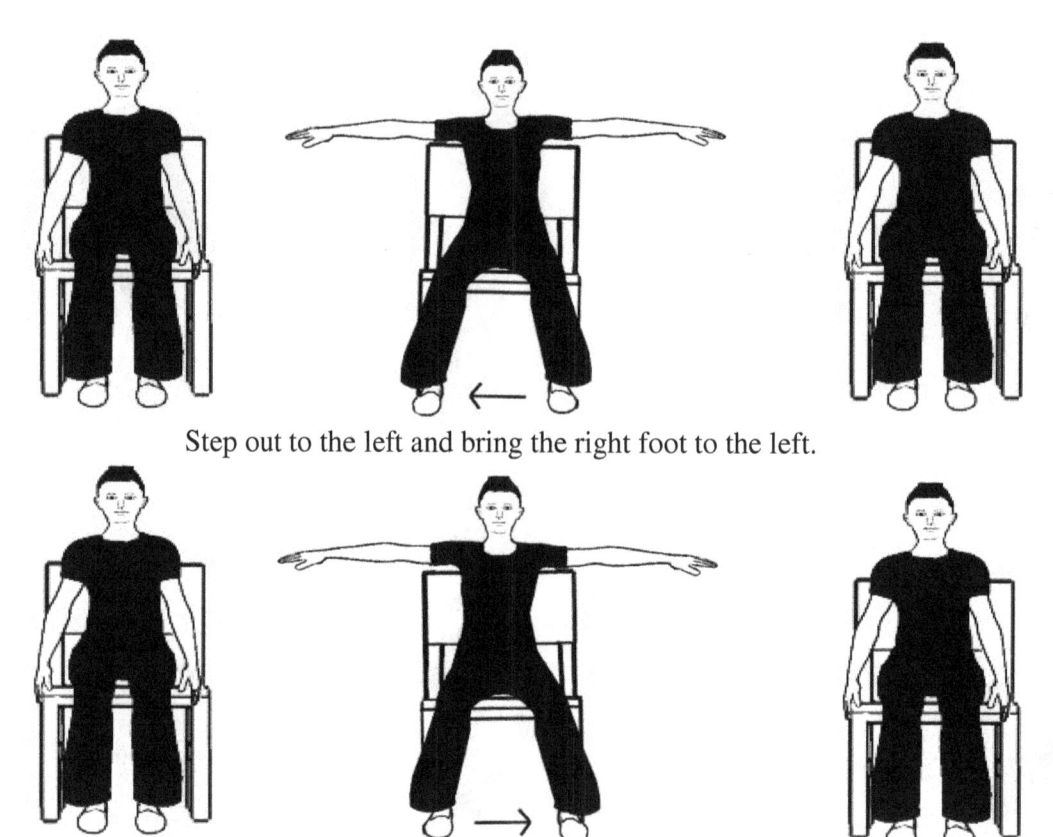

Step out to the left and bring the right foot to the left.

Continue stepping from right to left. Try to swing the arms up to shoulder height.

### Checklist
- Stand or sit up straight. Think of pushing the crown of the head up to the ceiling without lifting the chin
- Do as much as you can standing without holding on
- Swing your arms up to shoulder height level
- Focus on taking as wide of a step as you can
- Periodically use the Rating of Perceived Exertion or talk test (pg. 46) to check if you are exercising at the right level
- Breathe

## Alternate Knee Lifts

Alternately lift your knees as high as you can while keeping your balance and your back straight. Swing the opposite arm to leg.

Standing

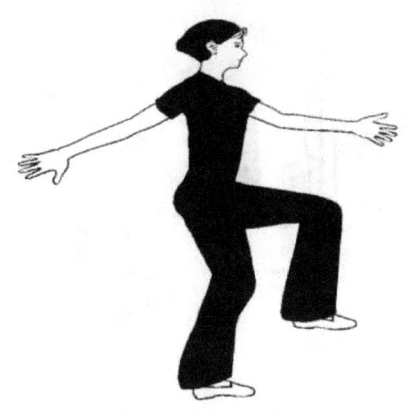

Standing with assistance

Do not lean on the chair or grab it too tight. Let your legs work to support you.

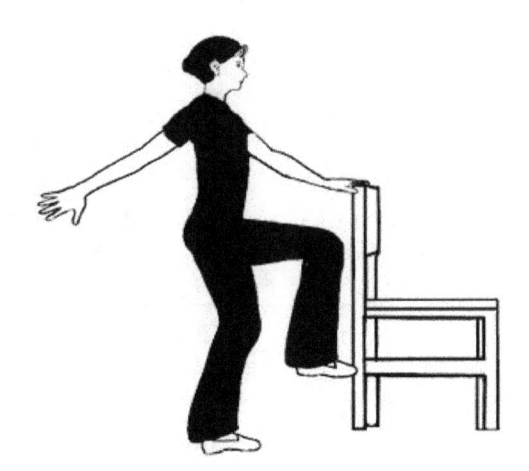

## Seated

You can also do alternate knee lifts while sitting in a chair. Sit up straight and away from the back of the chair as much as possible.

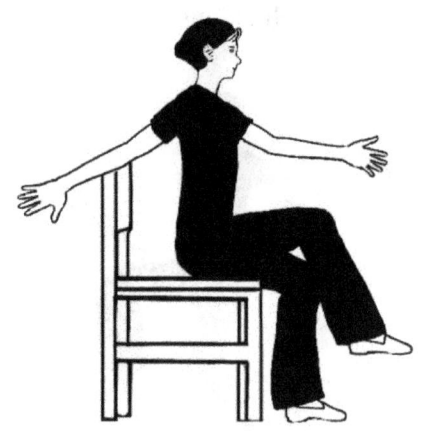

### Checklist
- ✓ Stand or sit up straight. Think of pushing the crown of the head up to the ceiling without lifting the chin
- ✓ Do as much as you can standing without holding on
- ✓ Swing your arms, using opposite arm to leg
- ✓ Try to avoid swinging the same arm as leg, which can bring you out of balance
- ✓ Focus on bringing the knee up to waist height if you can
- ✓ Periodically use the Rating of Perceived Exertion or talk test (pg. 46) to check if you are exercising at the right level
- ✓ Breathe

## Alternate Heel Curls Back

Alternately lift your heels to the back as high as you can, keeping your balance and your back straight. Swing the opposite arm forward.

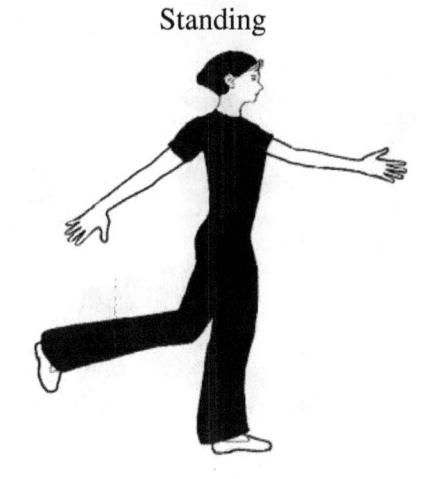

### Standing

### Standing with assistance
Do not lean on the chair or grab it tightly. Let your legs work to support you.

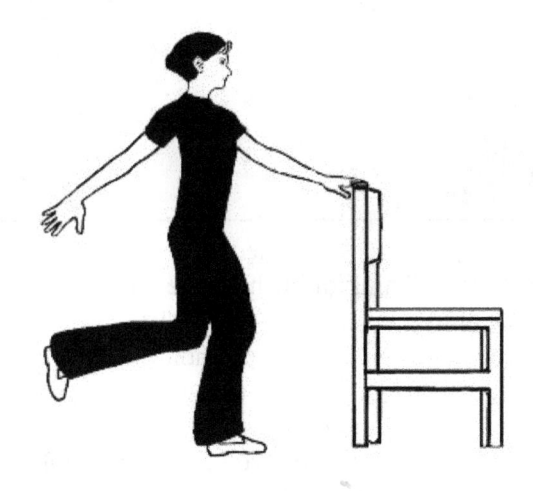

Seated

You can also do alternate heel curls while sitting in a chair. Sit up straight and away from the back of the chair as much as possible.

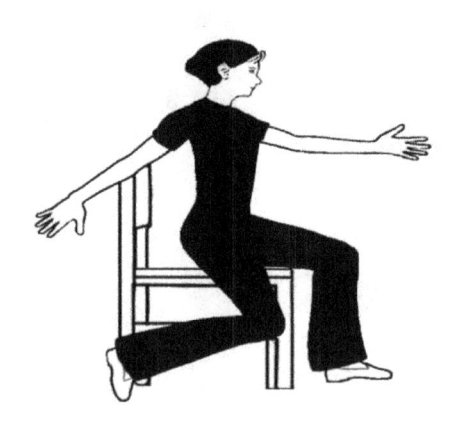

---

### Checklist
- ✓ Stand or sit up straight. Think of pushing the crown of the head up to the ceiling without lifting the chin
- ✓ Do as much as you can standing without holding on
- ✓ Swing your arms, using opposite arm to leg
- ✓ Focus on bringing the heel up to the back as high as you can
- ✓ Periodically use the Rating of Perceived Exertion or talk test (pg. 46) to check if you are exercising at the right level
- ✓ Breathe

## Side Toe Tap

Reach the right toe directly out to the side, as the arms lift up to the side. Do not put any weight on the toe. Keep your weight in the left leg. Bring the right leg back to the center.

Reach the left toe directly out to the side, as the arms lift up to the side. Do not put any weight on the toe. Keep your weight in the right leg. Bring the left leg back to the center.

Standing

Tap the right toe to the side, reaching the arms out.   Comeback to center.   Tap the left toe to the side, reaching the arms out.

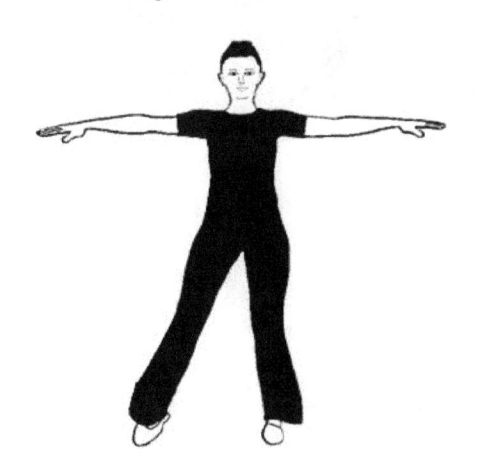

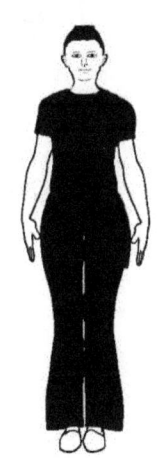

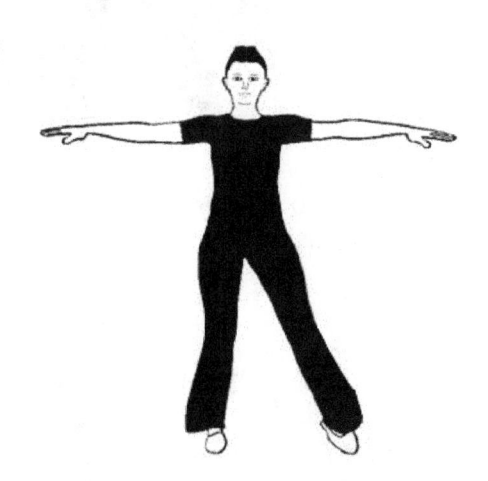

Continue alternating from side to side.

## Standing with assistance
Do not lean on the chair or counter or grab it too tightly. Let your legs work to support you.

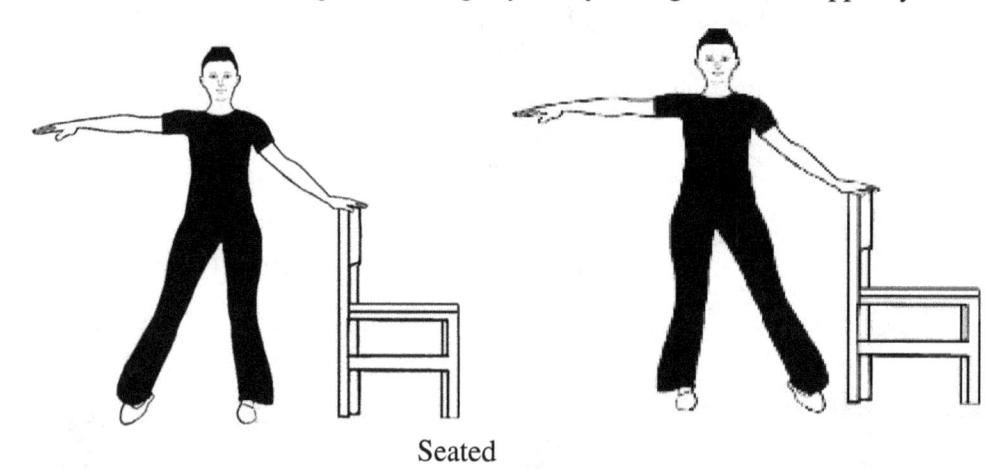

## Seated
You can also do alternate side toe taps while sitting in a chair. Sit up straight and away from the back of the chair as much as possible.

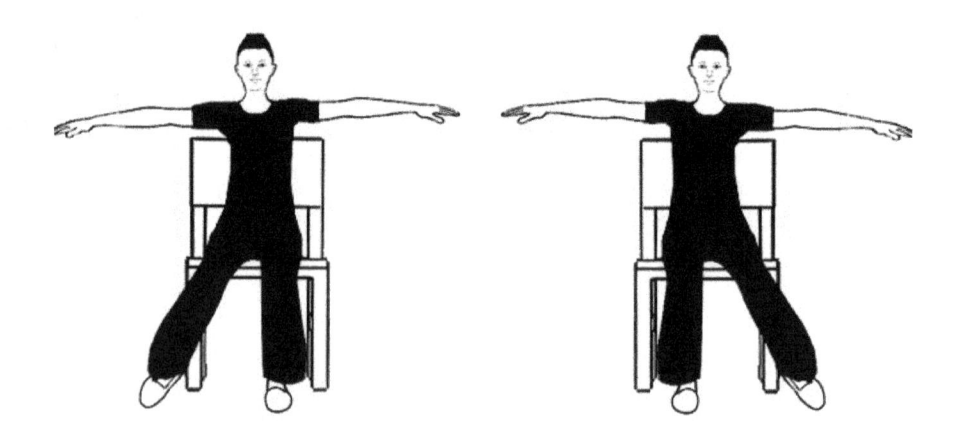

### Checklist
- Stand or sit up straight. Think of pushing the crown of the head up to the ceiling without lifting the chin
- Do as much as you can standing without holding on
- Swing your arms, trying to bring them shoulder height
- Reach the toe directly out to the side as far as you can without putting any weight in the toe
- Face forward through this movement. Do not twist the back or knees
- Periodically use the Rating of Perceived Exertion or talk test (pg. 46) to check if you are exercising at the right level
- Breathe

**Alternate Forward Heel Taps**
Flex the foot and tap just the heel of the foot on the ground in front of you.
Do not place the whole foot on the floor, or put any weight on the front foot.
Alternately tap heels in front. Swing opposite arm to foot.

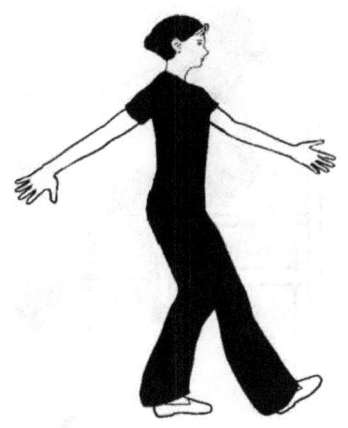

Standing

Standing with assistance
Do not lean on the chair or grab it too tightly. Let your legs work to support you.

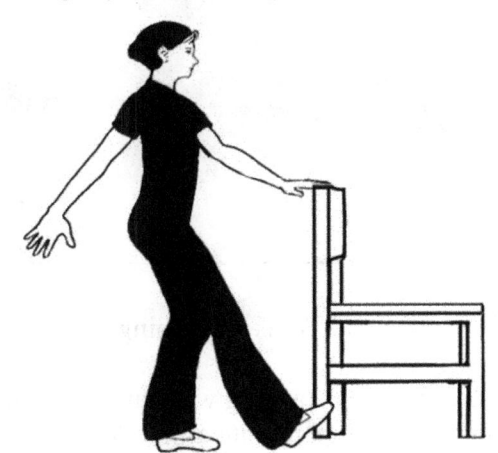

## Seated

You can also do alternate heel taps seated in a chair. Sit up straight and away from the back of the chair as much as possible.

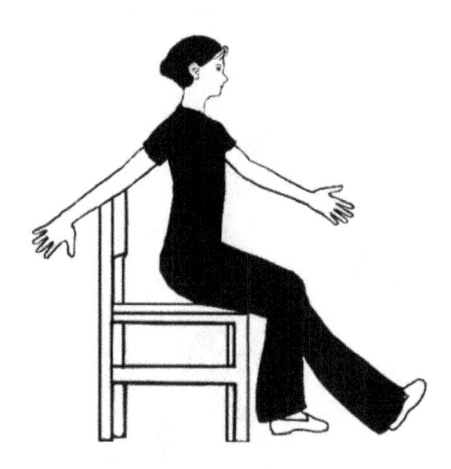

### Checklist

- ✓ Stand or sit up straight. Think of pushing the crown of the head up to the ceiling without lifting the chin
- ✓ Do as much as you can standing without holding on
- ✓ Swing your arms, using opposite arm to leg
- ✓ Try to avoid swinging the same arm as leg, which can bring you out of balance
- ✓ Focus on touching just the heel on the floor and keeping your weight in your back leg
- ✓ Periodically use the Rating of Perceived Exertion or talk test (pg. 46) to check if you are exercising at the right level
- ✓ Breathe

## Low Impact Jumping Jacks

Stand up straight and bring the arms up to shoulder height. Step the right foot out wide and squat, bringing the arms overhead. Make sure you keep equal weight in both legs as you squat down. To avoid knee injury do not lunge to the side. Bring the right foot back to the center. Then step out and squat with the left foot. Continue side to side.

Standing

Step out and squat right.          Comeback to center.          Step out and squat left.

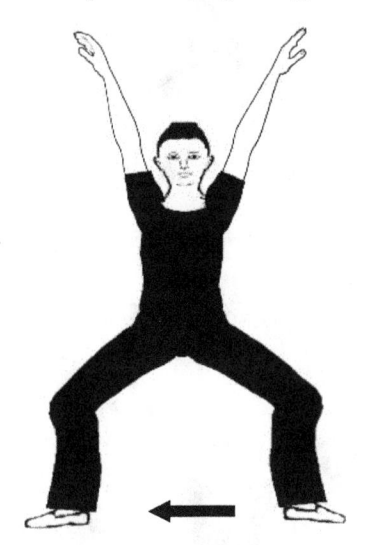

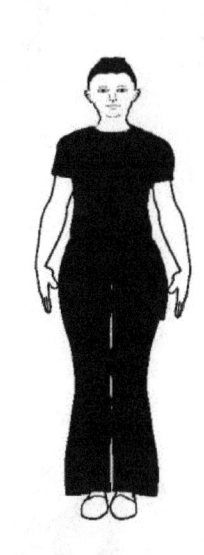

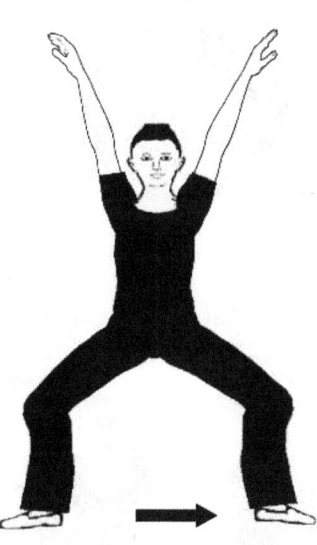

## Standing with Assistance
Do not lean on the chair or grab it too tightly. Let your legs work to support you.

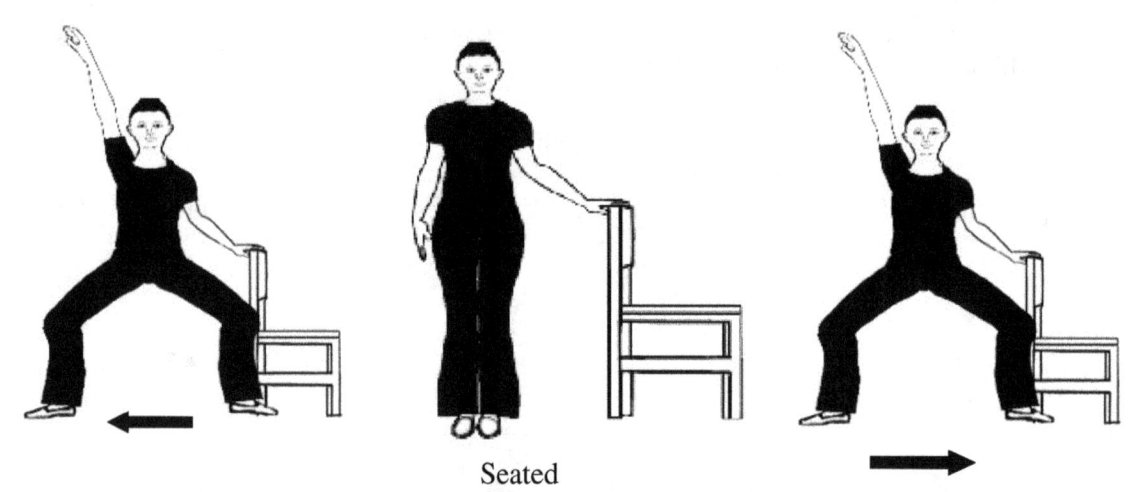

## Seated
You can also do jumping jack seated in a chair.
Sit up straight and away from the back of the chair as much as possible.

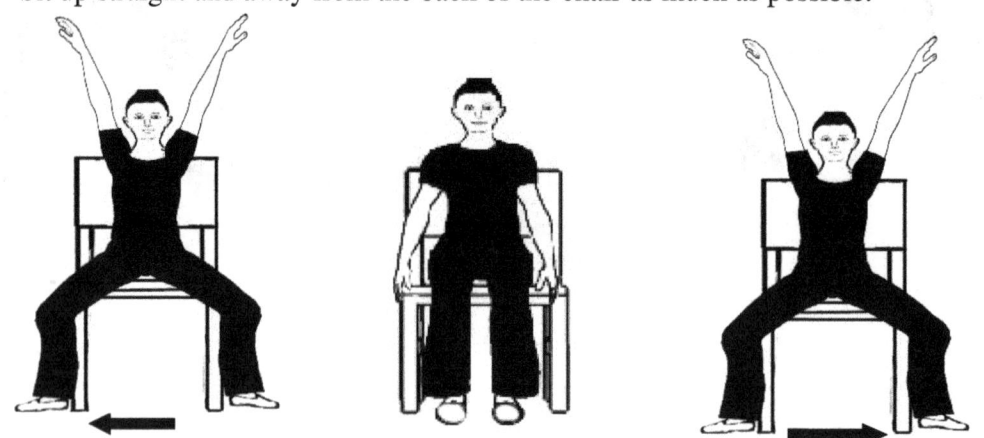

### Checklist
- ✔ Stand or sit up straight. Think of pushing the crown of the head up to the ceiling without lifting the chin
- ✔ Do as much as you can standing without holding on
- ✔ Swing your arms up overhead or as high as you are able
- ✔ Focus on landing with equal weight in both feet and avoid lunging to one side.
- ✔ Periodically use the Rating of Perceived Exertion or talk test (pg. 46) to check if you are exercising at the right level
- ✔ Breathe

## Lunges

Stand up straight. Step the right foot out straight in front of you and lift the arms up to shoulder height. Bend the left knee and drop straight down. Then push off the front foot and bring the right foot back to center. Next, step forward with the left foot and then bring the left foot back. Continue to alternate side to side. As you step forward keep the front knee aligned over the front ankle. Make sure you drop straight down and do not lunge forward as this can injure the knee.

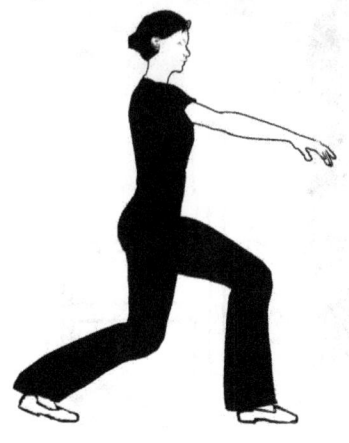

Standing

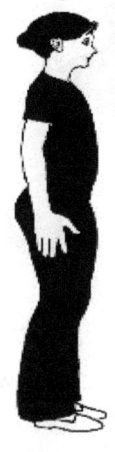

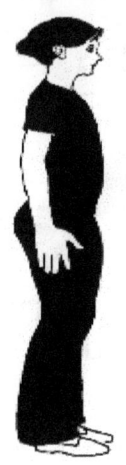

Step the right foot forward.                Bring the right foot back.

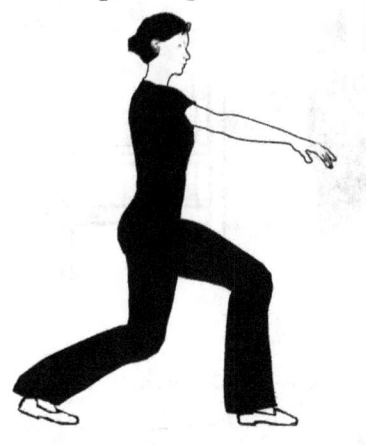

Step the left foot forward.                 Bring the left foot back

## Standing with assistance
Do not lean on the chair or grab it too tightly. Let your legs work to support you.

Step the right foot forward.

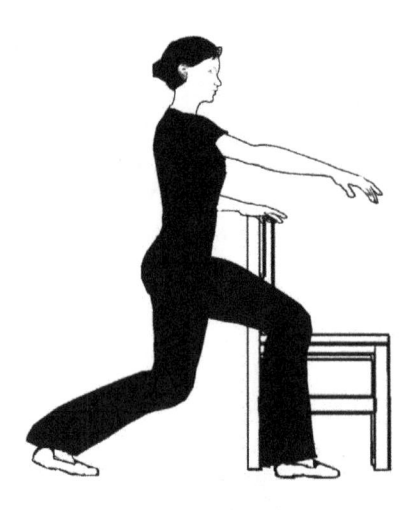

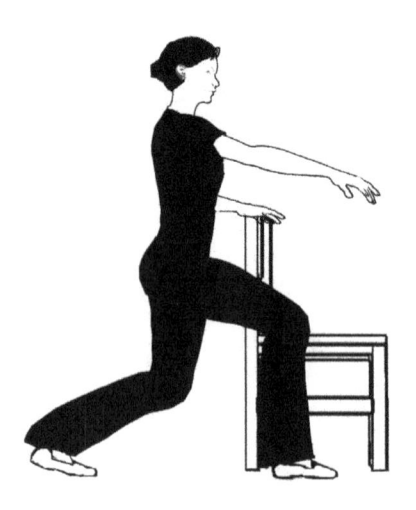

Bring the right foot back.

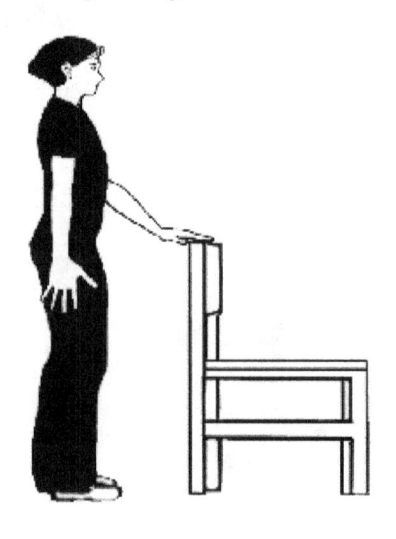

Step the left foot forward.

Bring the left foot back.

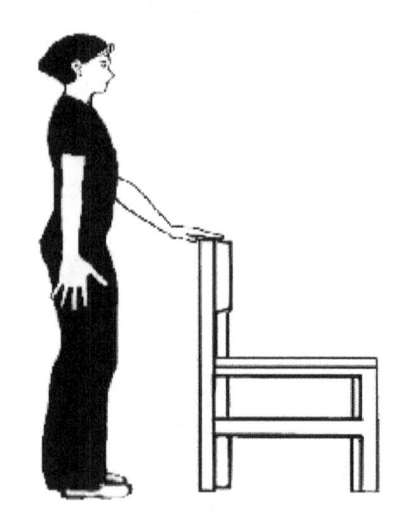

## Seated
You can also do lunges seated in a chair.
Sit up straight and away from the back of the chair as much as possible.

Step the right foot forward.

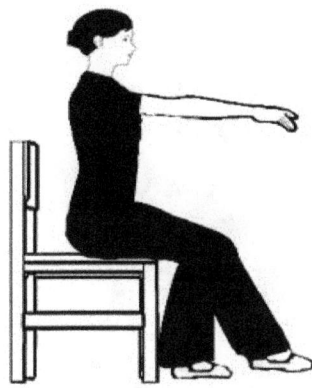

Bring the right foot back.

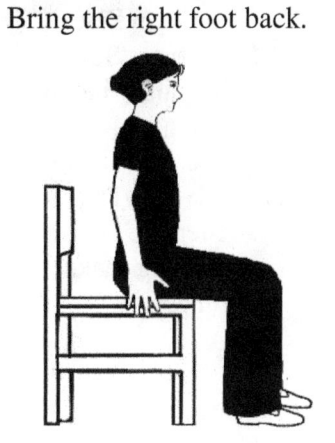

Step the left foot forward.

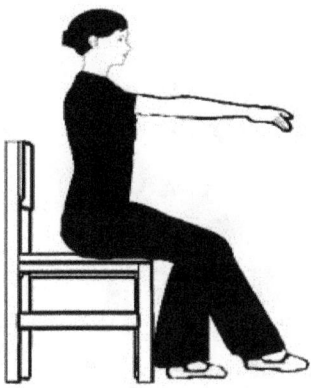

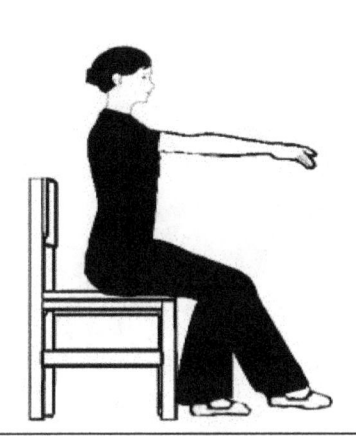

Bring the left foot back.

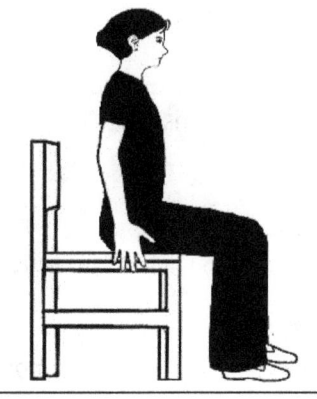

### Checklist
- Stand or sit up straight. Think of pushing the crown of the head up to the ceiling without lifting the chin
- Do as much as you can standing without holding on
- Swing your arms up to shoulder height.
- Focus on keeping the front knee over the front ankle and avoid lunging forward.
- Periodically use the Rating of Perceived Exertion or talk test (pg. 46) to check if you are exercising at the right level
- Breathe

# Putting It All Together

Start with three to five minutes of rhythmic limbering exercises or a short walk.

>March in Place.
>Alternate Straight Leg Kicks.
>Stepping Side to Side.
>Alternate Knee Lifts.
>Alternate Heel Curls Back.
>Side Toe Tap.
>Alternate Forward Heel Taps.
>Jumping Jacks
>Lunges

## The 4 1/2 Minute Workout.

March in Place .... 30 seconds
Alternate Straight Leg Kicks .... 30 seconds
Stepping Side to Side.... 30 seconds
Alternate Knee Lifts.... 30 seconds
Alternate Heel Curls Back.... 30 seconds
Side Toe Tap.... 30 seconds
Heel Taps.... 30 seconds
Jumping Jacks ............ 30 seconds
Lunges ............ 30 seconds

## The 8 Minute Workout.

March in Place .... 60 seconds
Alternate Straight Leg Kicks .... 60 seconds
Stepping Side to Side.... 60 seconds
Alternate Knee Lifts.... 60 seconds
Alternate Heel Curls Back.... 60 seconds
Side Toe Tap.... 60 seconds
Heel Taps.... 60 seconds
Jumping Jacks ............ 60 seconds
Lunges ............ 60 seconds

## The 13 Minute Workout.

March in Place …. 1 minute 30 seconds
Alternate Straight Leg Kicks … 1 minute 30 seconds
Stepping Side to Side…. 1 minute 30 seconds
Alternate Knee Lifts…. 1 minute 30 seconds
Alternate Heel Curls Back…. 1 minute 30 seconds
Side Toe Tap…. 1 minute 30 seconds
Heel Taps….. 1 minute 30 seconds
Jumping Jacks…..1 minute 30 seconds
Lunges …….. 1 minute 30 seconds

## The 18 Minute Workout.

March in Place …. 2 minutes
Alternate Straight Leg Kicks … 2 minutes
Stepping Side to Side…. 2 minutes
Alternate Knee Lifts…. 2 minutes
Alternate Heel Curls Back…. 2 minutes
Side Toe Tap…. 2 minutes
Heel Tap …... 2 minutes
Jumping Jacks…..2 minutes
Lunges …….. 2 minutes

---

### Checklist
- Try creating your own sequence of movements to make up your aerobic workout
- Try moving around the room; march forward for 8, march back for 8, or when side stepping, travel 4 steps right then 4 steps left, etc.
- Remember the object is to keep moving, and to keep the heart rate up
- Try incorporating your favorite music into your routine
- Start slowly and build up gradually so your body can adapt
- Listen to your body to determine the appropriate level for each day
- Remember to use the Rating of Perceived Exertion or talk test (pg. 46) to check if you are exercising at the right level
- Breathe

# Chapter Four

## Strength Training

*I am only one, but I am one. I cannot do everything, but I can do something.
And I will not let what I cannot do interfere with what I can do.*
- Edward Everett Hale

Strength training or resistance training is another important component of an exercise program for those with osteoporosis. As the muscles become stronger, certain tasks such as standing, walking, rising from a chair, climbing stairs, and lifting objects becomes easier. Strength training or resistance training simply means performing movements against some kind of resistance. Such resistance can be your own body weight, free weights such as hand and ankle weights, theraband or tubing, or machines typically found at gyms. When beginning a strength training routine, it is advisable to have the guidance of an instructor to make sure you are performing the movements correctly. Aside from this you can get a complete and beneficial strength training workout at home.

Benefits of strength training include:
- Stronger muscles that can do bigger jobs (such as lifting heavier objects)
- Stronger muscles that will work longer before becoming exhausted
- Increase in lean body mass (more muscle, less fat)
- Increase in metabolism meaning more calories burned even at rest
- Increase in bone mineral density (stronger bones)
- Improvements in overall stability and balance
- Lower blood sugar levels
- Decrease in body fat
- Fewer body aches and less fatigue

If you have access to hand and ankle weights, this book will show you how to use them. However, when beginning an exercise routine you should use light weights. You will find that you will be able to increase the weight fairly quickly in the beginning. Eventually you will find a weight which you will use for a while. If you do not have weights at home you can use common household items to start, and wait to buy weights when you are ready for more resistance. Instead of hand weights try using full soup cans or cylinder-shaped plastic containers filled with water or sand. Plastic shampoo, milk bottles, or laundry detergent containers work well. For ankle weights you can substitute with an old pair of socks filled with sand to the appropriate weight. These can and then be tied or fastened with Velcro around your ankles.

How Much Weight Should You Use?

   Most people in our classes start with three pound weights. We suggest only doing 8-12 repetitions of each exercise, so this weight should be good for most. Using less may not give you enough resistance to gain strength. Using less weight with more repetitions does not provide as effective results. One way to help determine the appropriate amount of weight to use is a technique known as the "10 Rep Max." This means finding the maximum amount of weight you can lift for 10 repetitions. For example, if you can lift three pounds more than 10 times with no difficulty and with good form, then that weight is too light for you. On the other hand if you can just about do 10 repetitions with good form with five pound weights before getting too tired to continue, than five pounds is a good weight for you to use. However if you are rehabilitating from an injury, check with your healthcare provider to determine if using weights is appropriate for your situation.

   *Never* sacrifice good lifting technique or range of motion for weight. If the weight is too heavy to allow you to do the exercise correctly through the full range of motion, do not use weight or switch to a lighter weight. If you cannot perform the full range of motion even without weight, check with your healthcare provider about seeing a physical or occupational therapist who can address the issue. It is essential for those with osteoporosis to do all they can to maintain as much range of motion in the joints as possible in order to remain active and independent.

Some tips to make your strength training routine safe and effective follow.
- Stop any exercise that causes pain.
- Perform all of the movements *slowly and with control.* Use a *" four thousand count"* to both lift and lower the weights.
- Practice good posture and body mechanics while doing the exercises.
- Exhale when lifting the weight and inhale while lowering the weight.
- Do not grip hand weights too tightly. This can cause a rise in blood pressure.
- Movements should be done with precision. Do not use rapid or "jerky" movements, and *avoid* just swing the weights or body through the movements.
- Do not perform strengthening exercises on the same muscles two days in a row. Your muscles need 48 hours after lifting to repair and recover. If you need or wish to split up your routine, try working your arms one day, and your legs the next, but you should not work the same muscles on two consecutive days.
- Perform 8-12 repetitions of each exercise.
- When you are able to perform 12 repetitions with no difficulty and with good form, increase the amount of weight by two to three pounds.
- If you are unable to perform the entire series of strengthening exercises at one time, you can split the routine doing certain exercises at different times throughout the day, or by working your legs one day and your arms the next day.
- You may find you need different weights for different exercises, i.e., five pound weights for larger muscles and three pound weights for the smaller muscles.
- *Always "warm-up" before lifting weights to avoid injury.*

## *How To Do These Exercises*

The leg exercises will be illustrated in both standing and seated positions. Do as much as you can standing. When standing, it is strongly recommended that you hold onto a chair or counter for support. For this section it is important to challenge yourself with the weight or resistance. By holding on you lessen your chances of a fall allowing you to fully focus on lifting the weight.

The upper body exercises will be illustrated in a seated position. This again reduces the risk for a fall, enabling you to focus on challenging yourself with weight. Also, when performing upper body exercises, it is sometimes easier to maintain a straight back while seated. Lifting weights while standing, especially with heavier weights, can often lead to arching the back or locking the knees in order to lift the weight.

Accompanying each exercise is a diagram highlighting the muscle or muscle group the exercise is targeting. Although most exercises utilize additional muscles that assist and stabilize movement, the diagrams highlight the primary muscle or muscle group each exercise is targeting. In general, when strength training, it is usually recommended to start with the largest muscles in your body first; i.e., your legs, and work down to the smaller muscles in your arms. However, if are working with some type of split routine or altering the workout, do what works best for you.

Remember to proceed slowly and use correct form. With all movements in this book, use your own judgment as to what is right for your body each day.

# Exploring Movement
## *Why I need to exercise my muscles*

Muscles are required in order to move the body. Our skeletal system can not move itself. Along with the muscles and bones, joints which provide flexible connections between the bones, are also required in order for movement to occur. In order to move we need the muscles, the bones and the joints.

### *Bones*

Think of your bones as levers, or a rigid bar that moves around a fulcrum, the fulcrum being the joint. Bones and muscles are connected to each other by tough cords of tissue called tendons.

### *Joints*

In simple terms, a joint is an area of the body where two or more bones are joined together using a network of muscles, tendons, ligaments, and cartilage. Your body has different kinds of joints. Some such as those in your knees, work like door hinges enabling you to move your lower leg forward and back. The joints in your neck enable bones to pivot so you can turn your head. Still other joints like those in your shoulders enable you to move your arms 360 degrees. The range of motion or flexibility of a joint is determined by the tightness of the ligaments, tendons, muscles, and the joint capsule surrounding that joint.

### *Muscles*

The human body contains over 600 muscles. Your ability to do tasks is in part determined by the strength of the muscles surrounding the joint to exert the force or power needed to move the joint. Skeletal muscles create movement by contracting or shortening and pulling on the bones to which they are attached. As the muscle shortens it pulls or draws one of the bones at the joint towards the other bone at that same joint. Muscles can only pull, they do not push. As a result, muscles work in pairs to create movement.

### *Muscle contractions*

Muscles move in response to signals from your nervous system and brain. Skeletal muscle contractions start either with a thought in the brain that you wish to move, or from an involuntary reflex such as when a sensory nerve detects pain from heat or injury. There is also a slight contraction and relaxation of skeletal muscles required for maintaining a balanced static posture, such as when standing or sitting.

*Review*

You have a thought that you would like to bend your elbow so you can pick up a cup and take a drink. Your brain sends signals through your nervous system to:
- Make the required muscle contract (biceps muscle shortens pulling and bending the elbow)
- Make the opposing muscles relax (the triceps muscle lengthens to allow the elbow to bend)
- Recruit other muscles in the arms and shoulders to stabilize the movement (so the cup can be lifted to your mouth without spilling)

So, it is important to maintain muscle strength if we wish to maintain full range of motion and complete everyday tasks.

# Strength Training Exercises
## Leg Extension *Muscles worked: Quadriceps (Front top of thigh)*
*(Rectus femoris, vastus lateralis, vastus medialis, and vastus intermedius).*

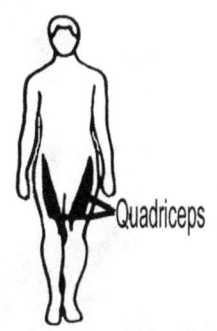

Before starting, check your posture. Stand up straight, bring the hips under the shoulders, and think about pushing the crown of the head to the ceiling without lifting the chin. Do 8-12 repetitions with the right leg, then 8-12 repetitions with the left leg.

### Standing

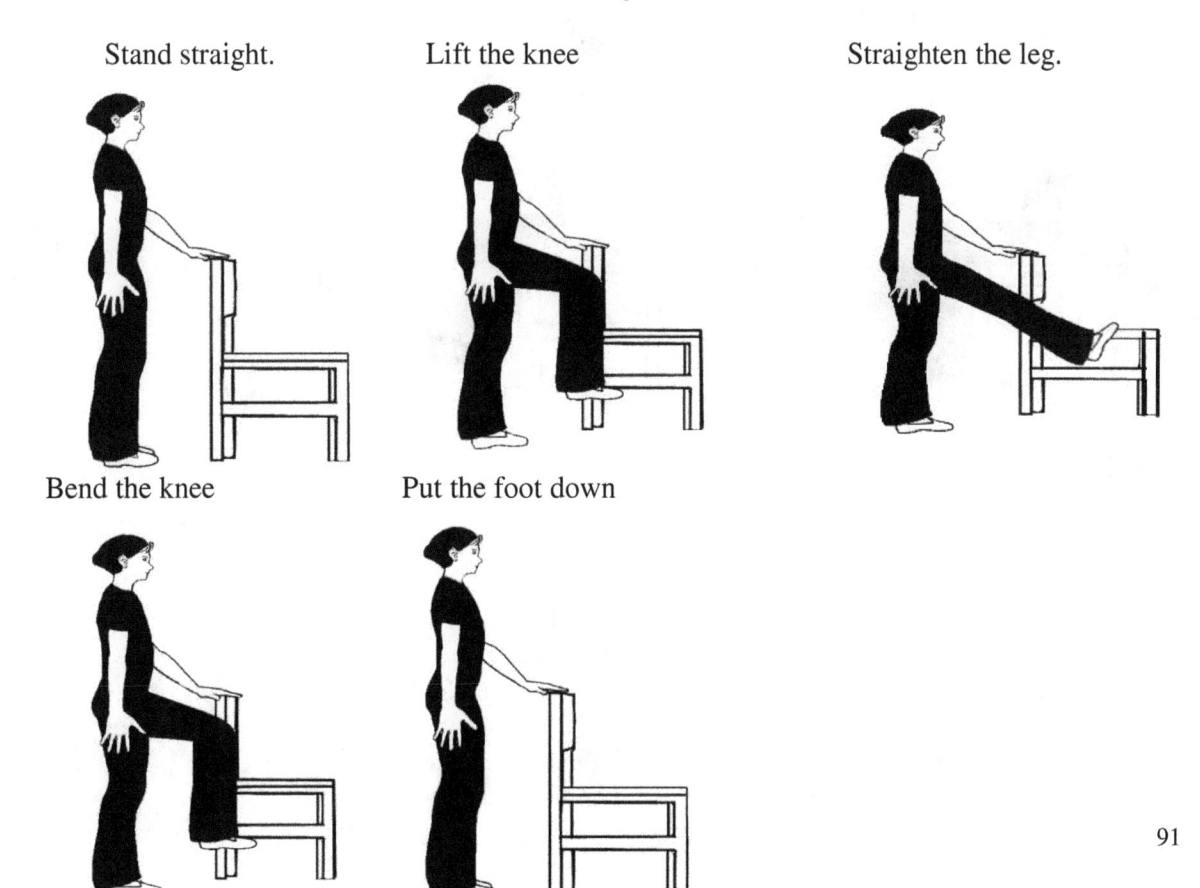

Stand straight.

Lift the knee

Straighten the leg.

Bend the knee

Put the foot down

91

## Seated

Sit up straight, away from the back of the chair if possible. If you need to sit back, sit all the way back to avoid slouching.

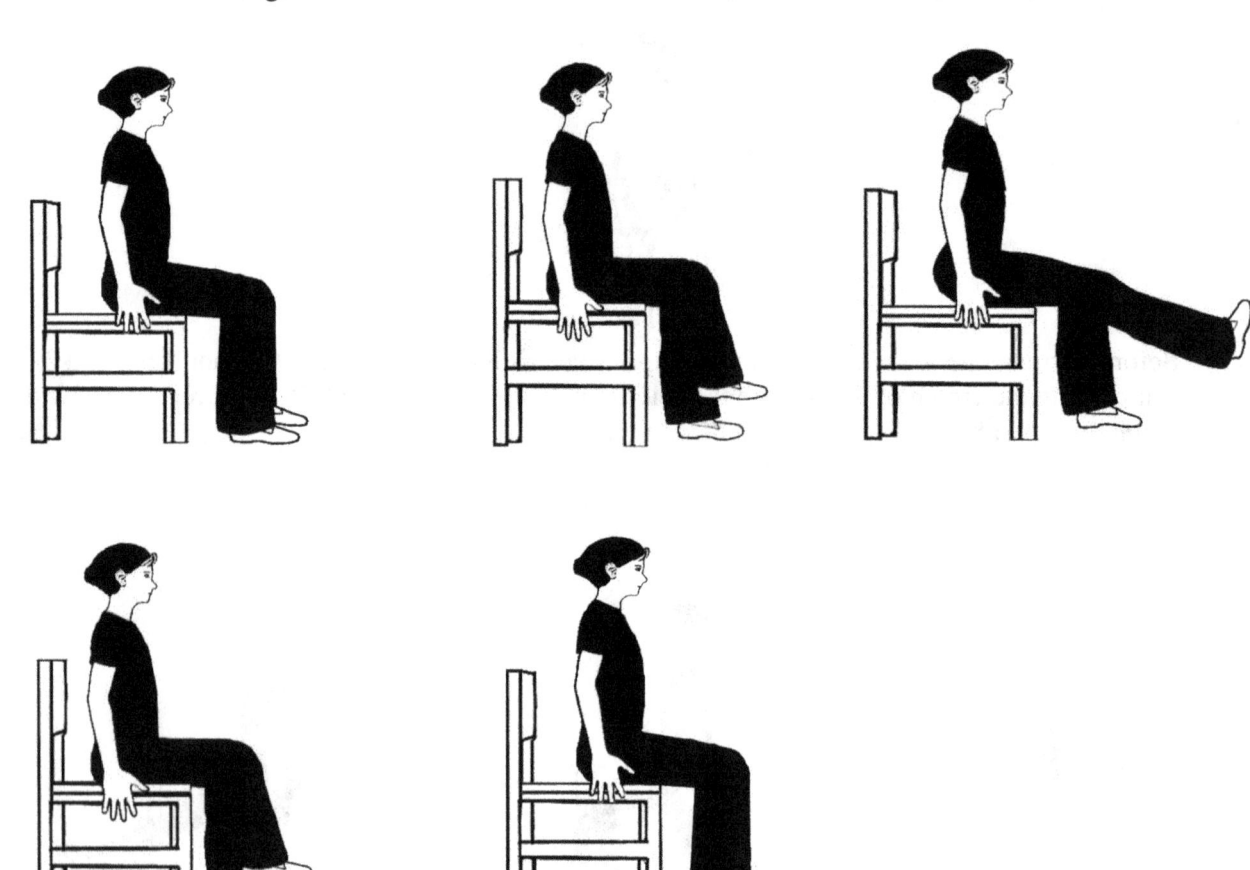

### Checklist

- ✓ Stand or sit up straight
- ✓ If possible do all repetitions on one leg and then switch to the other leg. If this bothers your hips or back you can alternate legs
- ✓ Move through your full range of motion, but do not lock the knee
- ✓ Ankle weights may be used if that feels appropriate
- ✓ Exhale as you lift the leg, inhale as you lower the leg
- ✓ Move slowly using a "4 thousand count" both to lift the leg and to lower the leg
- ✓ Use diaphragmatic breathing through the nose as much as possible
- ✓ Do not exercise to the point of strain or discomfort

**Squats**  *Muscles worked: Quadriceps (Front top of thigh)*
*(Rectus femoris, vastus lateralis, vastus medialis, and vastus intermedius).*

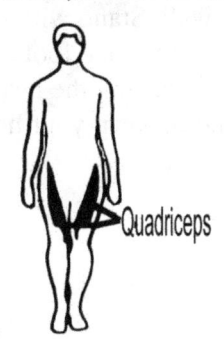

Before starting, check your posture. Stand up straight, bring the hips under the shoulders, and think about pushing the crown of the head to the ceiling without lifting the chin.

Have a chair behind you. Bring your arms up in front of you to chest height, with the palms facing the floor. Allow the natural curve in the low back to remain throughout this movement. Begin to bend your knees and reach your buttocks back as if you were going to sit in the chair. If able, lower the buttocks until they are parallel with your knees, and your knees are at a 90-degree angle. You may come into contact with the chair, but try not to sit all the way. If you can not go that far, just go as far as you are able. If your knees are sensitive, use caution with this movement. You will find that as your legs become stronger you will be able to go lower. Keep the weight forward and in your toes. This helps balance the body and prevents you from falling backwards. Make sure you do not lock the knees when you come back up to standing. Repeat 8-12 times.

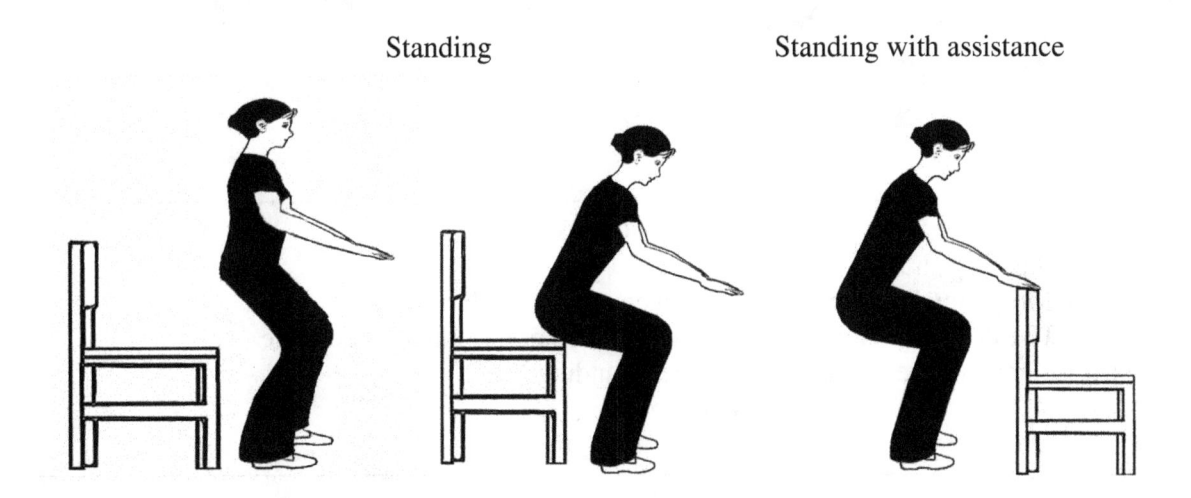

Standing                    Standing with assistance

## Against a wall

This movement can also be done against a wall. Stand with the hips, back, (including the low back) and shoulders against a wall. The feet can be about one foot away from the wall. Bring your head against the wall as well, if the head can touch keeping the head neutral without lifting the chin. Slide down no lower than a 45-degree angle and hold. Keep your heels on the floor.

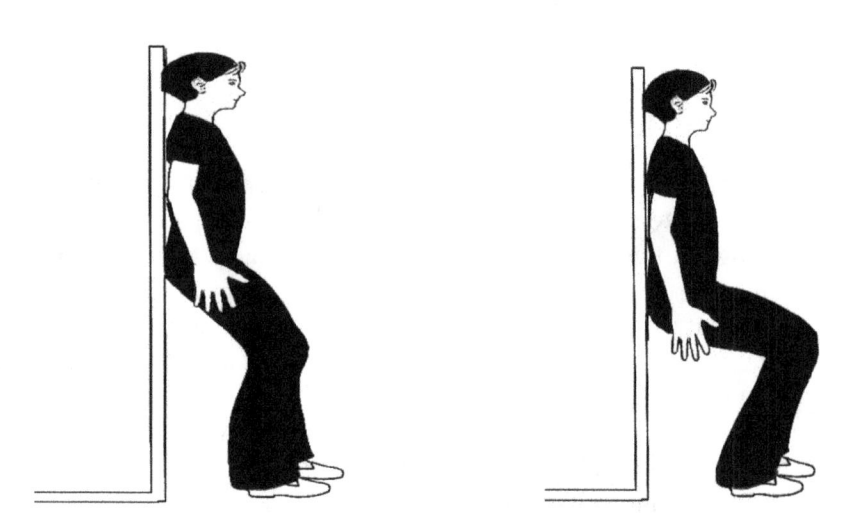

### Checklist
- ✓ Stand up straight
- ✓ Move slowly using a "4 thousand count" for each movement
- ✓ Use diaphragmatic breathing through the nose as much as possible
- ✓ Keep the knees slightly bent when standing
- ✓ Keep the natural arch in the low back
- ✓ Do not exercise to the point of strain or discomfort

**Side Leg Lift**   *Muscles worked: Abductors (Hip, outer thigh)*
*(Tensor fasciae late, gluteus medius, and gluteus minimus)*

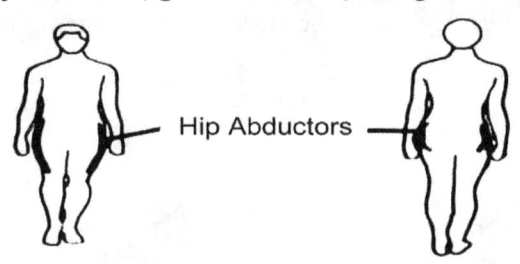

Hip Abductors

Standing

Before starting, check your posture. Stand up straight, bring the hips under the shoulders, and think about pushing the crown of the head to the ceiling without lifting the chin. Lift the leg straight out to the side. Do 8-12 repetitions with the right leg, then 8-12 repetitions with the left leg. Let the heel lead with the toes facing forward. *Do not let the leg turn out.*

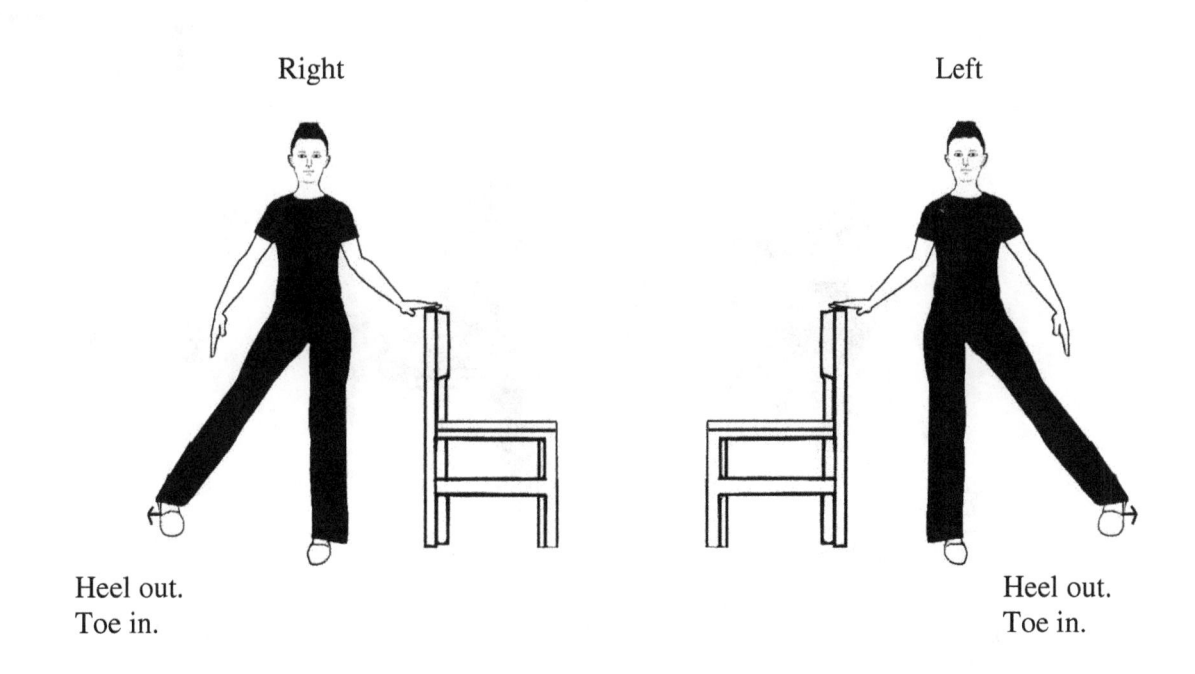

Right                                                           Left

Heel out.                                                       Heel out.
Toe in.                                                         Toe in.

## Seated

Sit up straight, away from the back of the chair if possible. If you need to sit back, sit all the way back to avoid slouching. Bring the leg out to the side without swinging the hips.

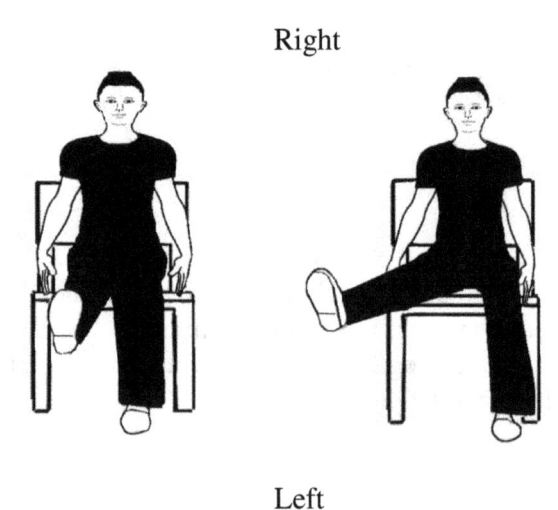

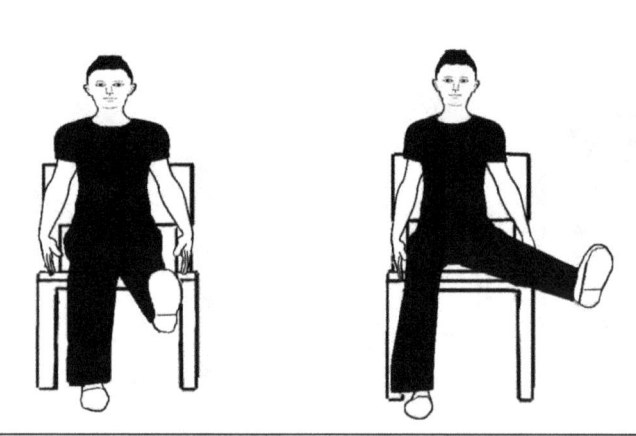

### Right

### Left

### Checklist

- ✓ Stand or sit up straight
- ✓ If possible do all repetitions on one leg and then switch to the other leg. If this bothers your hips or back you can alternate legs
- ✓ Move through your full range of motion, but do not swing the hips, or tip the shoulders
- ✓ Ankle weights may be used if that feels appropriate
- ✓ Exhale as you lift the leg, inhale as you lower the leg
- ✓ Move slowly using a "4 thousand count" both to lift the leg and to lower the leg
- ✓ Use diaphragmatic breathing through the nose as much as possible
- ✓ Do not exercise to the point of strain or discomfort

# Standing Leg Lift Back and Seated Heel Curl
*Muscles worked: Gluteal & Hamstring Muscles (Buttocks, back top of thigh)*
*(Gluteus maximus, biceps femoris, semitendinosus, and semimembranosus)*

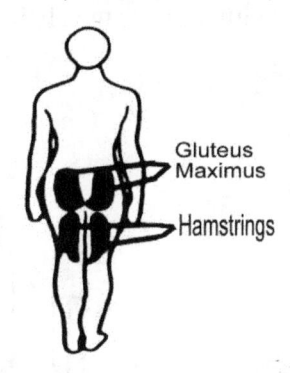

Before starting, check your posture. Stand up straight, bring the hips under the shoulders, and think about pushing the crown of the head to the ceiling without lifting the chin. Do 8-12 repetitions with the right leg, then 8-12 repetitions with the left leg.

## Standing Leg Lift Back

Stand straight. Tighten the buttocks muscles. Lift the leg directly out to the back. Do not let the leg go out to the side. Do not let the shoulders tip forward.

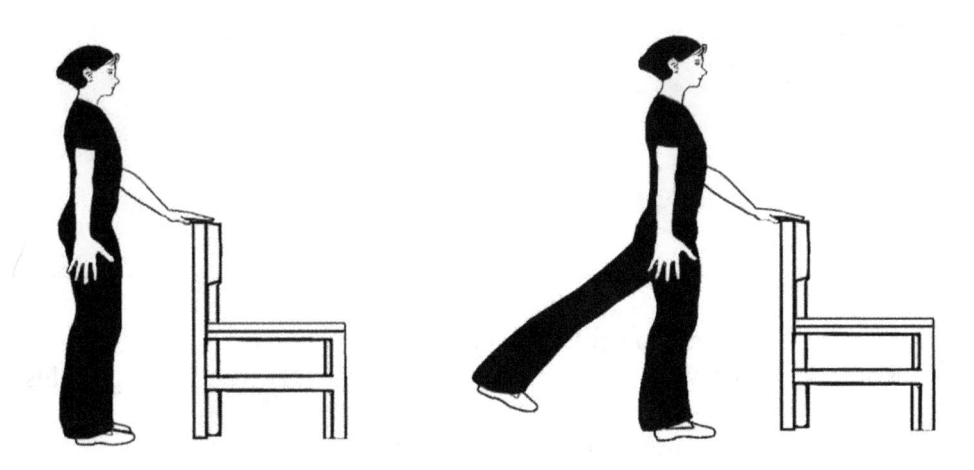

## Seated Heel Curl

Sit up straight, away from the back of the chair if possible. If you need to sit back, sit all the way back to avoid slouching. Pull the heel either under the chair or to the side depending on which is more comfortable for the knees.

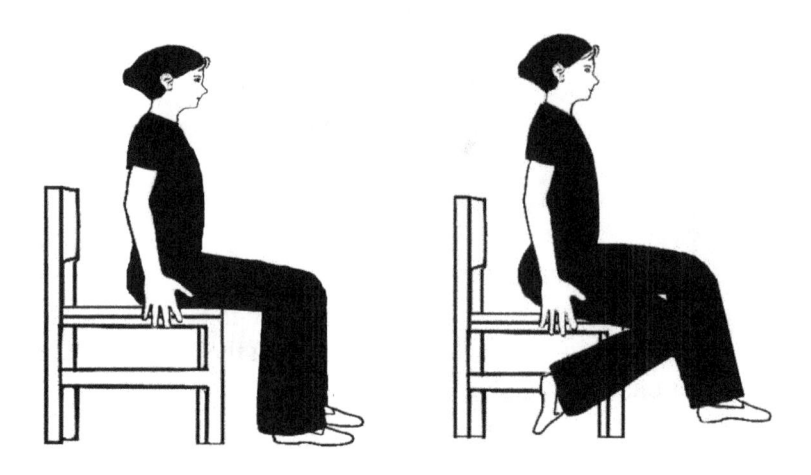

### Checklist
- ✓ Stand or sit up straight. Do not let the shoulders tip forward
- ✓ If possible do all repetitions on one leg and then switch to the other leg. If this bothers your hips or back you can alternate legs
- ✓ Ankle weights may be used if that feels appropriate
- ✓ Exhale as you bring the leg back, inhale as you bring the leg forward
- ✓ Move slowly using a "4 thousand count" both to lift the leg and to lower the leg
- ✓ Use diaphragmatic breathing through the nose as much as possible
- ✓ Do not exercise to the point of strain or discomfort

**Leg Crossover** *Muscles worked: Adductor Muscles (Inner thigh)*
*(Adductor longus, adductor brevis, and adductor magnus)*

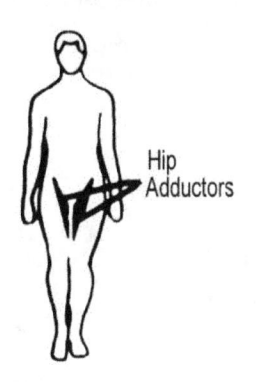

Standing

Before starting, check your posture. Stand up straight, bring the hips under the shoulders, and think about pushing the crown of the head to the ceiling without lifting the chin. Bring your leg in front and across your body. Let the knee bend and think about lifting your heel up. Do 8-12 repetitions with the right leg, then 8-12 repetitions with the left leg.

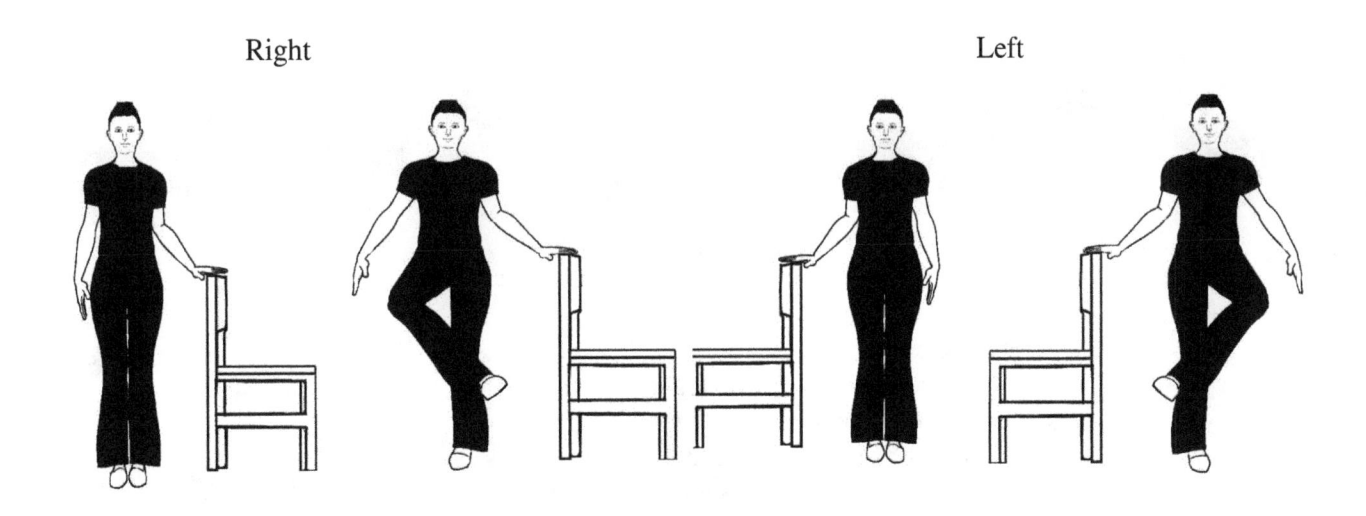

Right

Left

## Seated

Sit up straight, away from the back of the chair if possible. If you need to sit back, sit all the way back to avoid slouching. Let the knee bend and think about lifting your heel up to the front.

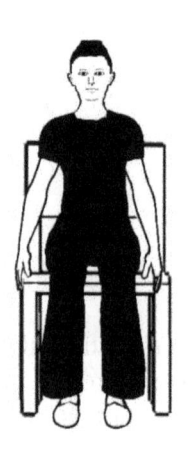

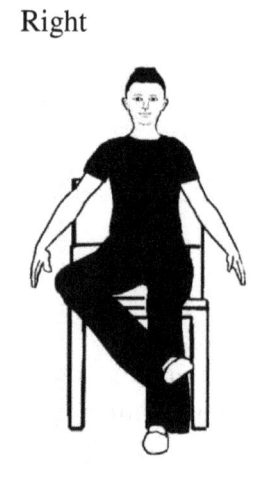

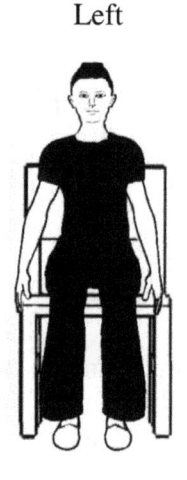

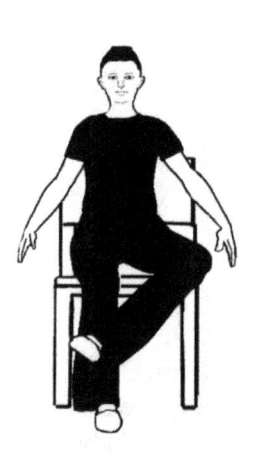

Right                    Left

### Checklist
- Stand or sit up straight
- If possible do all repetitions on one leg and then switch to the other leg. If this bothers your hips or back you can alternate legs
- Ankle weights may be used if that feels appropriate
- Exhale as you lift the leg, inhale as you lower the leg
- Move slowly using a "4 thousand count" both to lift the leg and to lower the leg
- Use diaphragmatic breathing through the nose as much as possible
- Do not exercise to the point of strain or discomfort

**Heel Raises**  *Muscles worked: Gastrocnemius and Soleus (Calf)*
*(Gastrocnemeus when standing and Soleus when seated)*

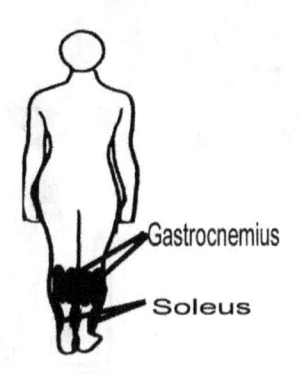

Standing

Before starting, check your posture. Stand up straight, bring the hips under the shoulders, and think about pushing the crown of the head to the ceiling without lifting the chin. Using the chair as little as possible, rise up onto the toes. When lowering just barely touch the heels, keeping most of the weight in the toes. Do 8-12 repetitions.

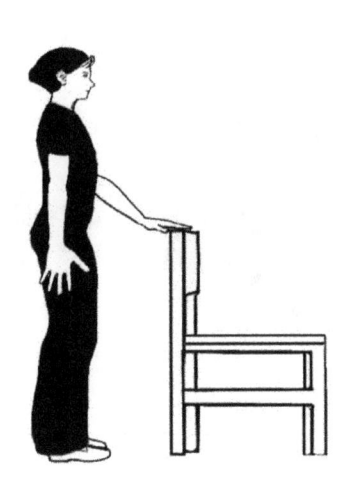

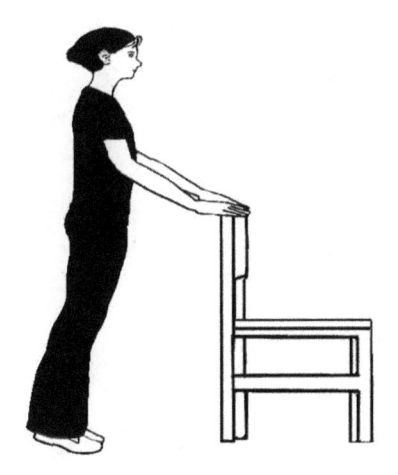

## Seated

Sit up straight, away from the back of the chair if possible. If you need to sit back, sit all the way back to avoid slouching.

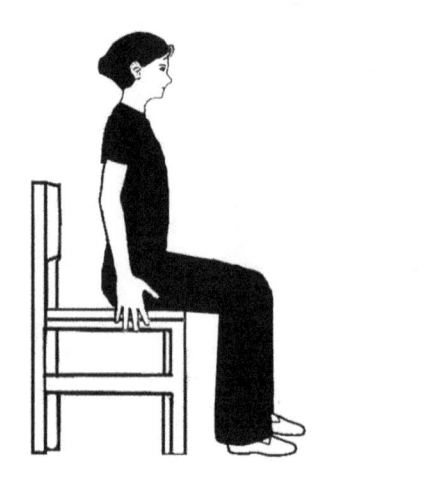

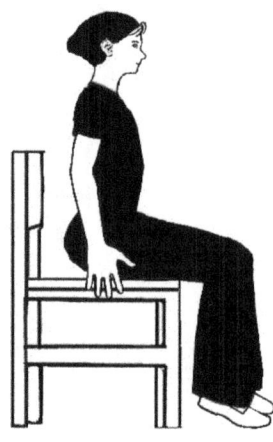

### Checklist
- ✓ Stand or sit up straight
- ✓ Ankle weights may be used if that feels appropriate
- ✓ Try to keep the weight in your toes and not back in your heels
- ✓ Move slowly using a "4 thousand count" both to lift the heels and to lower the heels
- ✓ Use diaphragmatic breathing through the nose as much as possible
- ✓ Do not exercise to the point of strain or discomfort

**Toe Lifts**
*Muscles worked: Tibialis Anterior (Shin)*

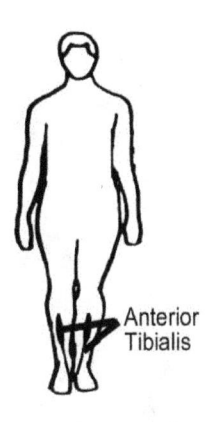

Before starting, check your posture. Stand up straight, bring the hips under the shoulders, and think about pushing the crown of the head to the ceiling without lifting the chin. Using the chair as little as possible, bend the knees slightly and lift up just the toes. Then lower slowly down. Make sure you do not rock the hips backwards and keep the heels down. Do eight to twelve repetitions.

Standing

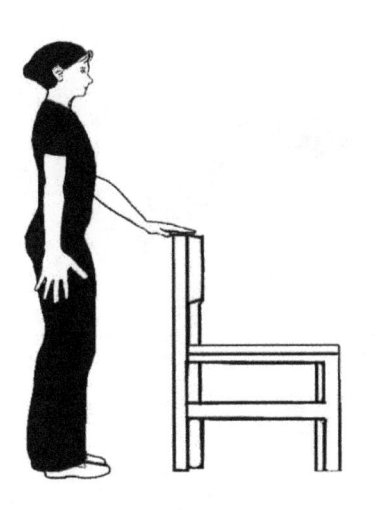

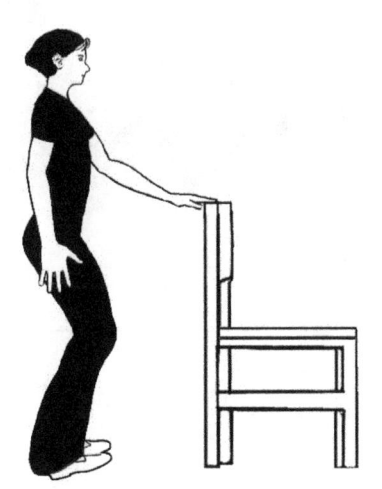

## Seated

Sit up straight, away from the back of the chair if possible. If you need to sit back, sit all the way back to avoid slouching.

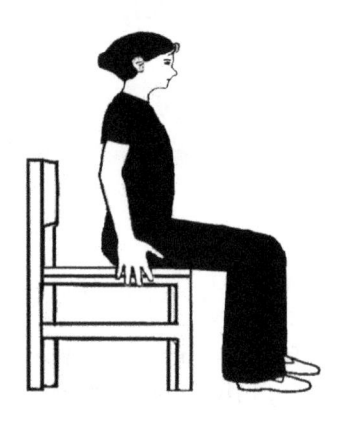

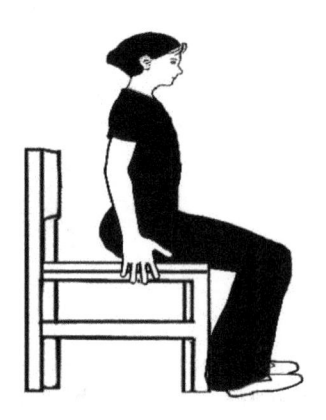

```
Checklist
✓  Stand or sit up straight
✓  Ankle weights may be used if that feels appropriate
✓  Move slowly using a "4 thousand count" both to lift the heels and to lower the heels
✓  Use diaphragmatic breathing through the nose as much as possible
✓  Do not exercise to the point of strain or discomfort
```

## Wall Pushups  *Muscles worked: Pectoralis Major (Chest)*

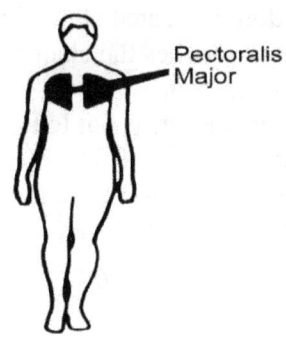

Stand arms-length away from the wall. Place your hands on the wall chest height and shoulder width apart. Bend the elbows and bring your nose and chest as close to the wall as possible, keeping your hips and shoulders in one line. Do not let your hips come forward. Do 8-12 repetitions.

Standing

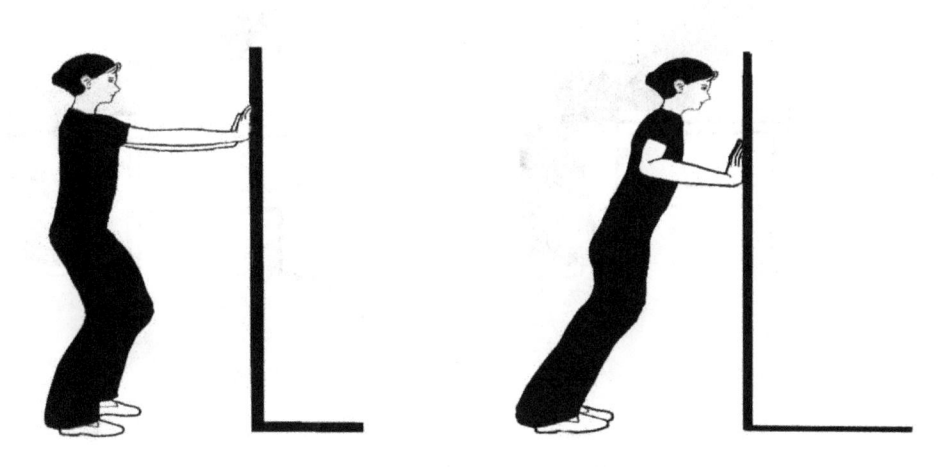

### Checklist
- ✓ Stand or sit up straight
- ✓ Do not lock the elbows
- ✓ Keep your body straight, do not let the hips and buttocks come forward
- ✓ Move slowly using a "4 thousand count" to both push away from the wall and to lower yourself towards the wall
- ✓ Exhale as you push away from the wall, inhale as you come to the wall
- ✓ Use diaphragmatic breathing through the nose as much as possible
- ✓ Do not exercise to the point of strain or discomfort

## Seated Chest Fly

You can work the same muscles by doing a seated chest fly. Sit at the very front edge of the chair. Then lean back so your upper back touches the chair for support. Do not drop your head back – keep your neck straight and in alignment.

*Keeping the elbows slightly bent,* open your arms out to the side. Do not let the wrists, hands or weights drop, make sure you control the movement. The bring the weights up in *front of your chest (not your face)* in a circular motion – like you were hugging something. Keep your elbows bent throughout this movement – both when opening the arms and lifting the arms. Exhale as you lift the weights, inhale as you lower them. Do eight to twelve repetitions.

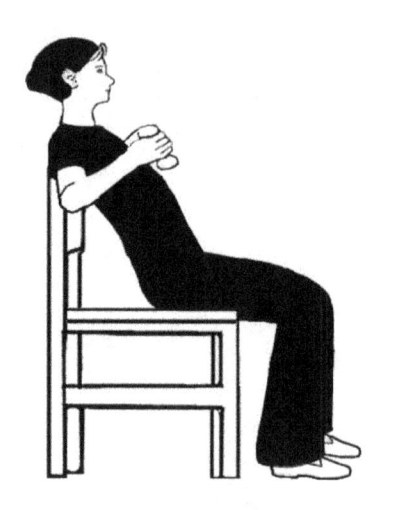

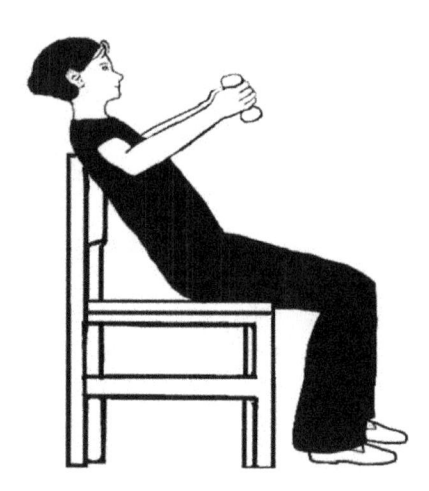

### Checklist
- Lean your upper back only against the back of the chair, keep the abdominal muscles tight to protect your back
- Do not lock the elbows
- Keep your arms rounded and the elbows bent throughout, do not drop the hands or wrists back
- Move slowly using a "4 thousand count" to both lift and lower the weights
- Exhale as you round forward, inhale as you open the arms
- Use diaphragmatic breathing through the nose as much as possible
- Do not exercise to the point of strain or discomfort

# Bent Row
*Muscles worked: Trapezius, Rhomboids, Latissimus Dorsi (Upper and mid back)*

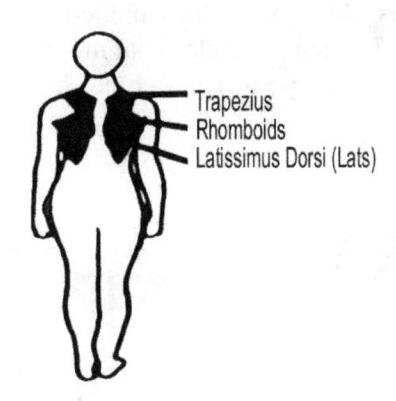

This exercise can be done seated or standing. The seated version may isolate the muscles better but it can place some strain on the back. Try both variations to see which version works best for you.

## Standing

In standing, this exercise is illustrated using just one arm at a time, to better isolate the muscles and to protect the back. Stand in a lunge position and place your left hand on the chair for support. Keep your arm and elbow close to your body and squeeze the shoulder blades together and lift the right elbow until your hand comes about waist height. Keep the abdominal muscles pulled in to protect the back. Do 8-12 repetitions with the right arm, then 8-12 repetitions with the left arm.

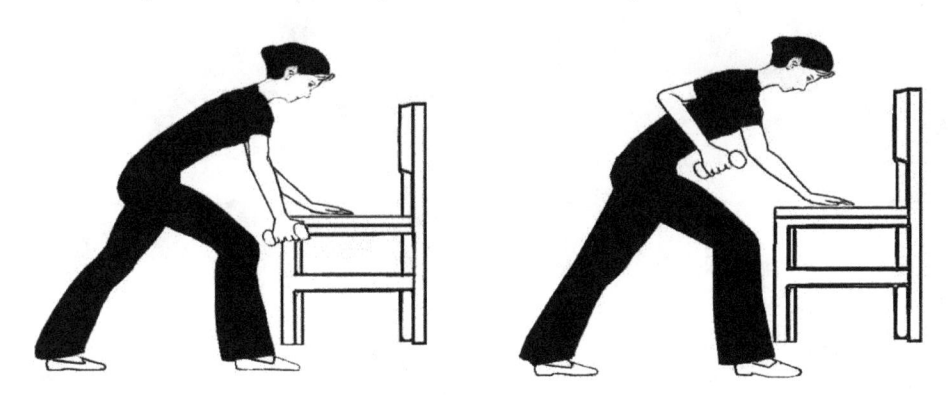

## Seated

For the seated version, lean forward from the hips and look down and slightly ahead. Do not lift the head and compress the neck. Tighten the abdominal muscles and squeeze the shoulder blades together as you lift both elbows up until your hands come about waist height. Do 8-12 repetitions.

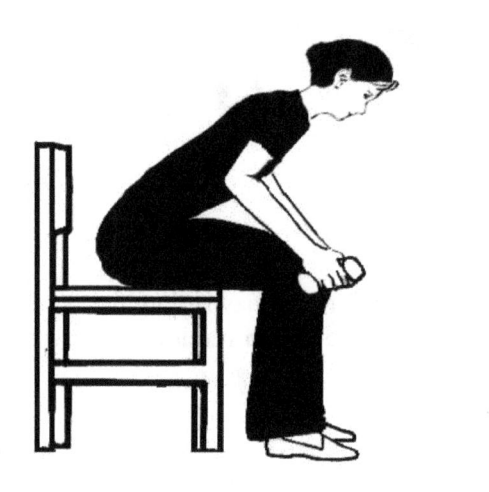

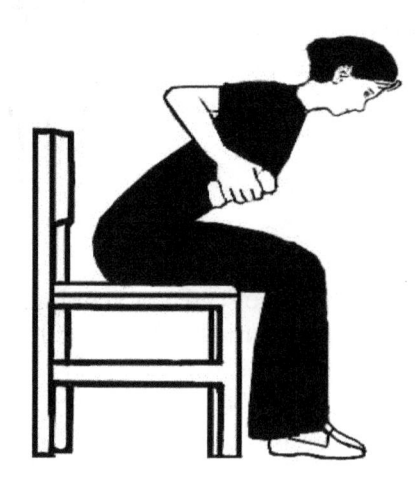

### Checklist
- ✓ Keep the abdominal muscles in and the back straight
- ✓ Do not lock the elbows
- ✓ Hand weights may be used if that feels appropriate
- ✓ Move slowly using a "4 thousand count" both to lift the weight and to lower the weight
- ✓ If using both arms at the same time bothers your back just do one arm at a time.
- ✓ Exhale as you lift the weight up, inhale as you lower the weight down
- ✓ Use diaphragmatic breathing through the nose as much as possible
- ✓ Do not exercise to the point of strain or discomfort

**Front Lateral Raise**  *Muscles worked: Deltoid (Shoulders)*

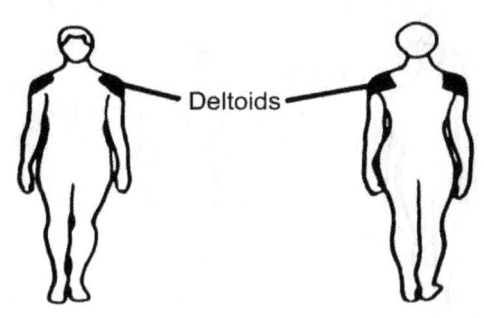

Before starting, check your posture. Sit at the front edge of the chair as much as possible in order to engage your abdominal muscles. If you need to sit back, sit all the way back in the chair to avoid slouching. Let the arms hang down at your sides with the palms facing back. Without rocking the body backwards lift the weights up in front of you to *shoulder height only*. Then lower slowly down. If lifting both arms at the same time bothers your back you can do just one arm at a time. Do 8-12 repetitions.

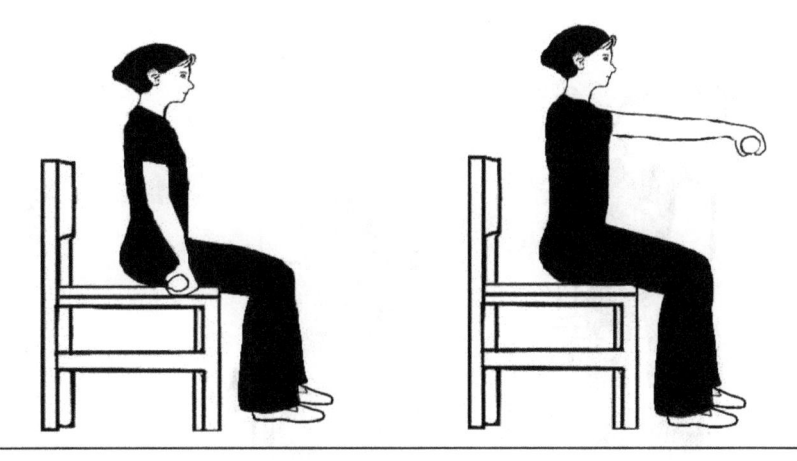

Checklist
- ✓ Sit up straight, away from the back of the chair if possible
- ✓ Hand weights may be used if that feels appropriate
- ✓ Exhale as you lift the weight up, inhale as you lower the weight
- ✓ Do not arch your back or rock backwards while lifting the weight
- ✓ Do not lock the elbows
- ✓ Make sure you only lift the weight to shoulder height
- ✓ Move slowly using a "4 thousand count" both to lift the weight and to lower the weight
- ✓ Use diaphragmatic breathing through the nose as much as possible
- ✓ Do not exercise to the point of strain or discomfort

## Military Press  *Muscles worked: Deltoid and Trapezius (Shoulders)*

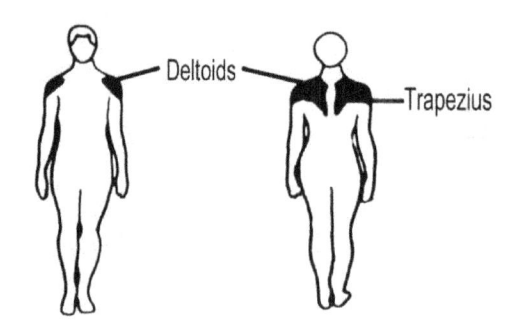

Before starting, check your posture. Sit at the front edge of the chair as much as possible in order to engage your abdominal muscles. If you need to sit back, sit all the way back in the chair to avoid slouching. Do 8-12 repetitions.

Bring your elbows to shoulder height. Turn your palms so they face forward instead of facing your ears as this helps to open the shoulders and prevent forward rounding of the shoulders. Bring the arms back towards the ears as much as possible. Exhale as you lift the weights straight up overhead. Try to straighten your elbows without locking them. Then lower slowly down until your elbows are at shoulder height again.

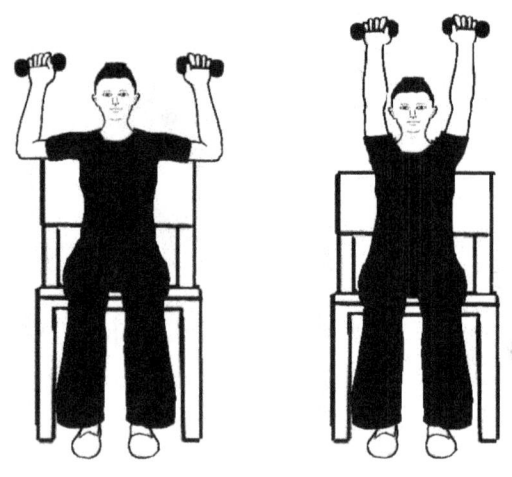

### Checklist
- ✓ Sit up straight, away from the back of the chair if possible
- ✓ Hand weights may be used if that feels appropriate
- ✓ Exhale as you lift the weight up, inhale as you lower the weight
- ✓ Do not arch your back or rock backwards while lifting the weight
- ✓ Do not lock the elbows
- ✓ Turn the hands so the palms face forward to avoid rounding the shoulders forward
- ✓ Move slowly using a "4 thousand count" both to lift the weight and to lower the weight
- ✓ Use diaphragmatic breathing through the nose as much as possible
- ✓ Do not exercise to the point of strain or discomfort

**Deltoid Raise**  *Muscles worked: Deltoid (Shoulders)*

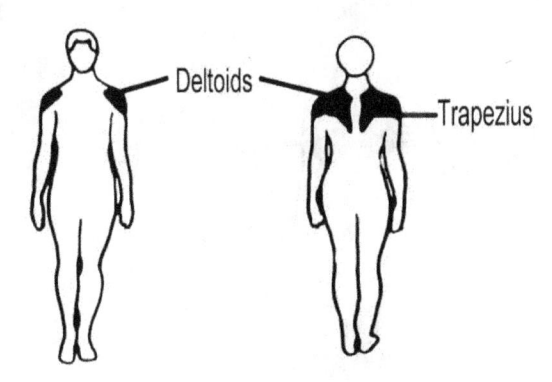

Before starting, check your posture. Sit at the front edge of the chair as much as possible in order to engage your abdominal muscles. If you need to sit back, sit all the way back in the chair to avoid slouching.

Bring your hands down by your side. Exhale as you lift straight up to the side, to shoulder height only. Your palms should be facing the floor. Keep your elbows straight but do not lock them. Then lower slowly down. Do 8-12 repetitions.

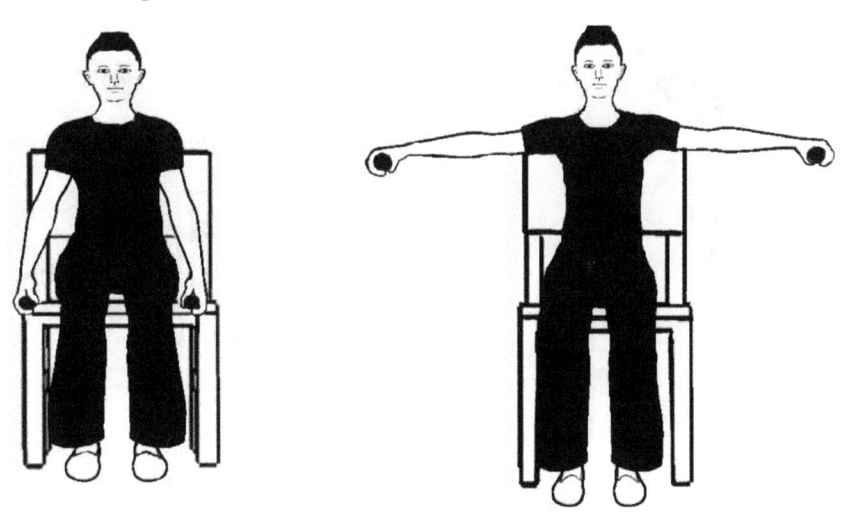

Checklist
- Sit up straight, away from the back of the chair if possible
- Hand weights may be used if that feels appropriate
- Exhale as you lift the weight up, inhale as you lower the weight
- Do not arch your back or rock backwards while lifting the weight
- Do not lock your elbows
- Move slowly using a "4 thousand count" both to lift the weight and to lower the weight
- Use diaphragmatic breathing through the nose as much as possible
- Do not exercise to the point of strain or discomfort

**Biceps Curl**  *Muscles worked: Biceps (Front top of arm)*

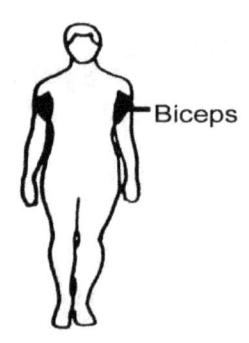

Before starting, check your posture. Sit at the front edge of the chair as much as possible in order to engage your abdominal muscles. If you need to sit back, sit all the way back in the chair to avoid slouching.

Bring your hands down by your side. Turn your palms so they face forward. Exhale as you bend your elbows, bringing the weights to your shoulders. Keep your elbows at your side. *Do not lift the elbows to bring the weight up.* Do 8-12 repetitions.

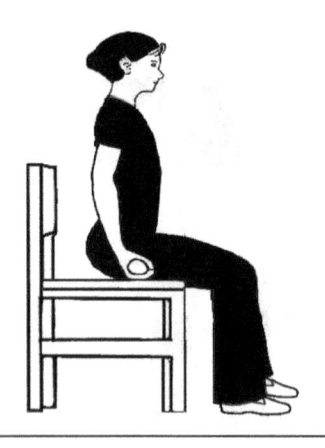

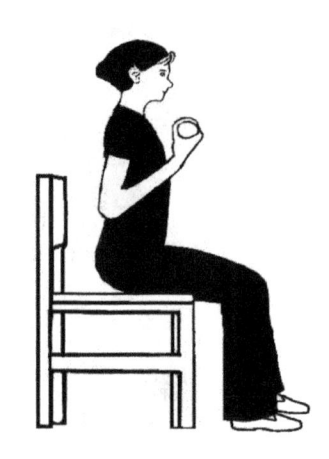

Checklist
- Sit up straight, away from the back of the chair if possible
- Hand weights may be used if that feels appropriate
- Exhale as you lift the weight up, inhale as you lower the weight
- Do not arch your back or rock backwards while lifting the weight
- Do not lock your elbows
- Move slowly using a "4 thousand count" both to lift the weight and to lower the weight
- Use diaphragmatic breathing through the nose as much as possible
- Do not exercise to the point of strain or discomfort

**Triceps Kickback**  *Muscles worked: Triceps (Back top of arm)*

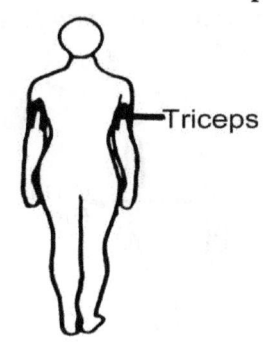

Before starting, check your posture. Sit at the front edge of the chair and tighten your abdominal muscles.

Bring your elbows to your sides and lean slightly forward without straining your back. Leaning forward helps to better isolate the muscle. Keep the abdominal muscles tight. Straighten your arms and bring the weights back. Then, just bend at the elbows to bring the hands back. Avoid swinging the whole arm. The movement is just at the elbow joint. If doing both arms at the same time bothers your back you can do just one arm at a time. Do 8-12 repetitions.

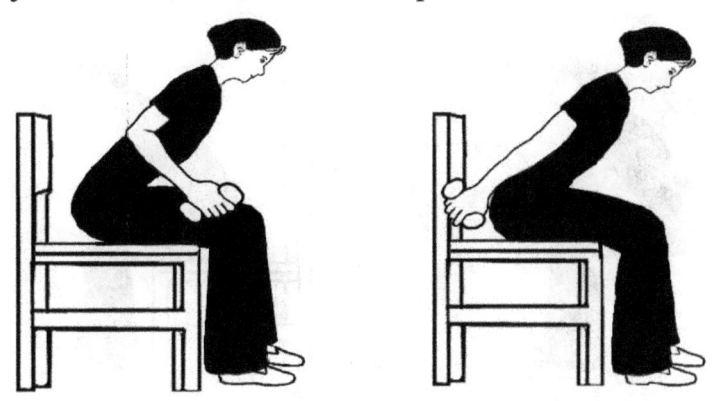

| Checklist |
| --- |
| ✓ Lean forward enough to better isolate the muscle, but not too far as to strain the back |
| ✓ Hand weights may be used if that feels appropriate |
| ✓ Exhale as you straighten the elbow, inhale as you bend the elbow |
| ✓ Do not swing your whole arm just bend and straighten the elbows |
| ✓ Do not lock your elbows |
| ✓ Move slowly using a "4 thousand count" both to straighten the elbow and to bend the elbow |
| ✓ Use diaphragmatic breathing through the nose as much as possible |
| ✓ Do not exercise to the point of strain or discomfort |

## Wrist Curls  *Muscles worked: Flexor Carpi Radialis, Flexor Carpi Ulnaris*
*(Front of wrists and forearm)*

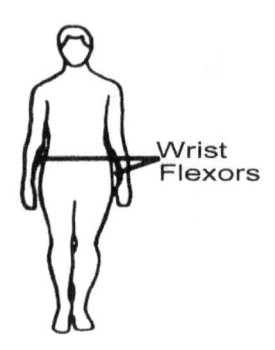

Before starting, check your posture. Sit at the front edge of the chair as much as possible in order to engage your abdominal muscles. If you need to sit back, sit all the way back in the chair to avoid slouching.

Lean forward placing the back of your wrists and elbows on your thighs. Your hands should be past your knee. Hold the weight with the palms facing the ceiling. Exhale as you curl the wrist up. Keep the movement in the wrist only, do not lift your arms off of your thighs. Do 8-12 repetitions.

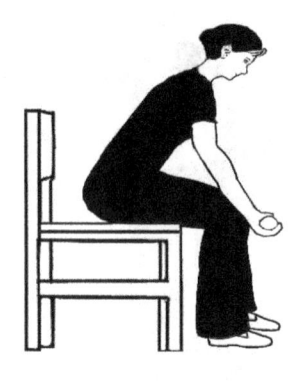

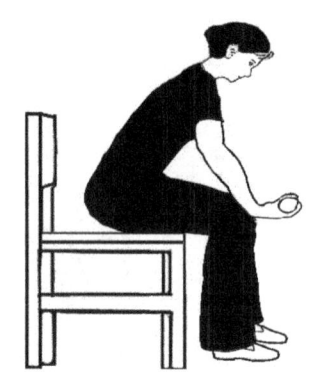

### Checklist
- ✓ Sit up straight, away from the back of the chair if possible
- ✓ Hand weights may be used if that feels appropriate
- ✓ Exhale as you lift the weight up, inhale as you lower the weight
- ✓ Do not lift your elbow or forearm off of your thigh, keep the movement just in the wrist
- ✓ Move slowly using a "4 thousand count" both to curl the wrist up and to lower the wrist
- ✓ Use diaphragmatic breathing through the nose as much as possible
- ✓ Do not exercise to the point of strain or discomfort

# Reverse Wrist Curls
*Muscles worked: Extensor Carpi Radialis Brevis, Extensor Carpi Ulnaris*
*(Back of wrists)*

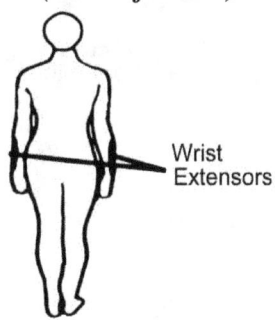

Before starting, check your posture. Sit at the front edge of the chair as much as possible in order to engage your abdominal muscles. If you need to sit back, sit all the way back in the chair to avoid slouching.

Lean forward placing the front of your wrists and elbows on your thighs. Your hands should be past your knee. Hold the weight with the palms facing the floor. Exhale as you curl the wrist up. Keep the movement in the wrist only, do not lift your arms off of your thighs. Do 8-12 repetitions.

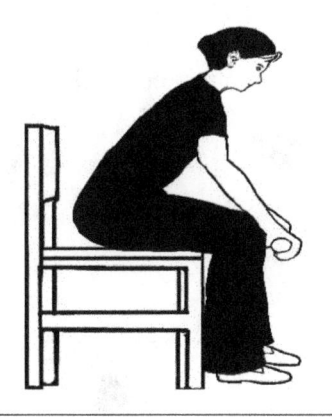

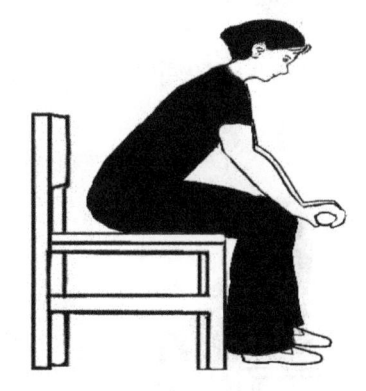

### Checklist
- Sit up straight, away from the back of the chair if possible
- Hand weights may be used if that feels appropriate
- Exhale as you lift the weight up, inhale as you lower the weight
- Do not lift your elbow or forearm off of your thigh, keep the movement just in the wrist
- Move slowly using a "4 thousand count" both to curl the wrist up and to lower the wrist
- Use diaphragmatic breathing through the nose as much as possible
- Do not exercise to the point of strain or discomfort

**Lean Backs**   *Muscles worked: Rectus Abdominus (Abdominal muscles)*

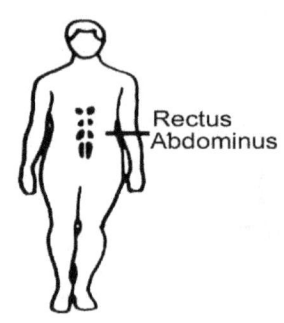

For this exercise you need to sit at the front edge of the chair so you have plenty of room to lean back.

Cross your arms at your chest. Inhale as you sit up straight letting the low back arch slightly. Exhale and tuck the chin into the chest. Let the low back round slightly and lean back. Go back far enough that you feel a pull in the abdominal muscles, but not so far that you touch the back of the chair. Make sure the back stays rounded. If you feel this exercise in your back instead of in the abdominal muscles, you may be arching your back. Keep the chin tucked, do not let your head drop back. Keep the shoulders down and relaxed. Hold back for a five-second count, make sure you do not hold your breath. Inhale and come back up straight. Do 8-12 repetitions.

Sit up, low back arched slightly.    Lean back, chin tucked, back rounded.

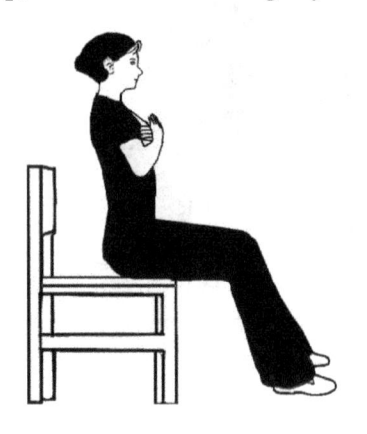

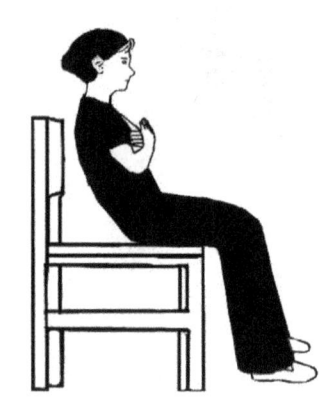

### Checklist
- ✓ Sit up straight, away from the back of the chair if possible
- ✓ Inhale as you sit up, exhale as you lean back
- ✓ Keep the spine slightly rounded
- ✓ Do not drop the head back, keep the chin tucked
- ✓ Move slowly using a "4 thousand count" both to lean back and to come forward
- ✓ Use diaphragmatic breathing through the nose as much as possible
- ✓ Do not exercise to the point of strain or discomfort

# Bicycles:
## *Muscles worked: Rectus Abdominus (Abdominal muscles)*

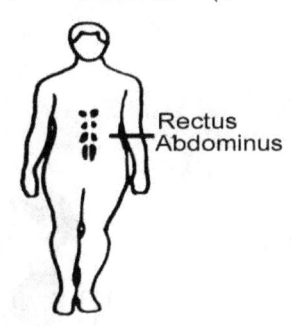

This exercise works the lower abdominal muscles. Before starting, check your posture. Sit at the front edge of the chair so you have room to lean back. Cross your arms at your chest. Inhale as you sit up and let the low back arch slightly. Tuck the chin into the chest, round the back and lean back. Go back until you feel a pull in the abdominal muscles without touching the chair. Keep your back rounded. If you feel this exercise in your back instead of in the stomach, you may be arching your back. Do not drop the head back and keep the shoulders down. Hold back as you lift either one leg at a time or bicycle the legs for a count of six times. Come back up and repeat. Do not hold your breath. Do five to six repetitions.

Sit up straight. Lean back alternately lifting legs.
This version is better for those with sensitive backs.

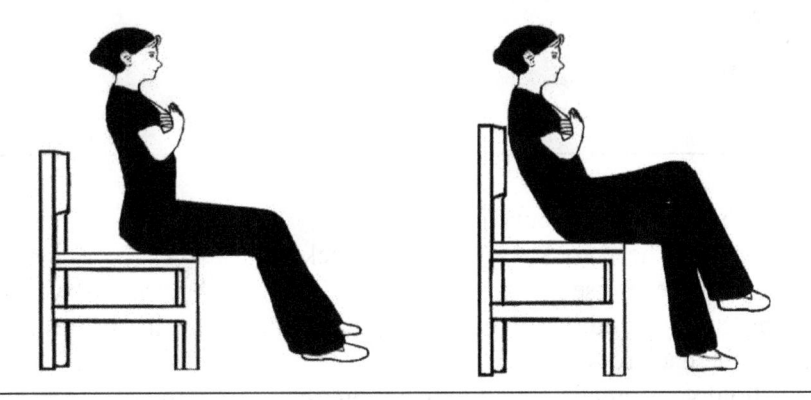

### Checklist
- ✓ Keep the spine slightly rounded and the chin tucked in
- ✓ Do not hold your breath. Breathe in and out throughout the exercise
- ✓ Use diaphragmatic breathing through the nose as much as possible
- ✓ Do not exercise to the point of strain or discomfort

Lean back and bicycle both legs about 5 to 6 times.
Repeat for 6 to 8 repetitions. This is a more challenging variation.

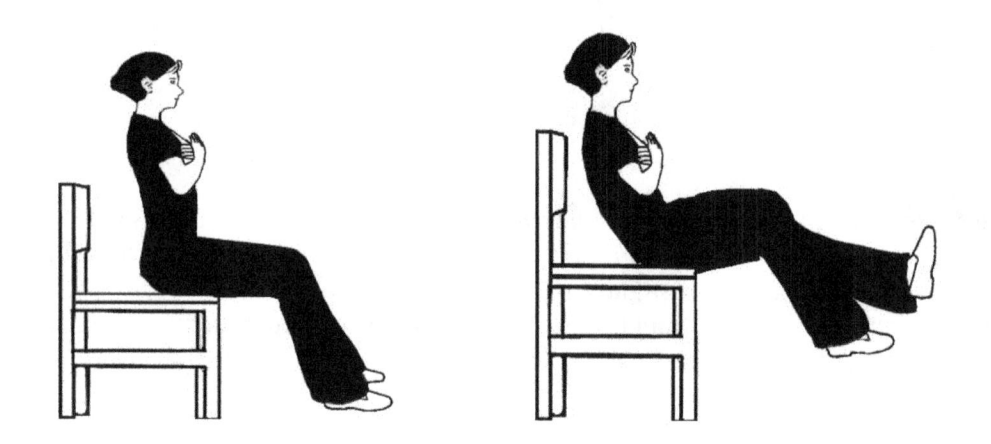

#### Checklist
- ✓ Keep the spine slightly rounded
- ✓ Do not drop the head back, keep the chin tucked
- ✓ If you feel this exercise in your back instead of your abdominals you are probably arching your back. Focus on pulling the stomach muscles in and keeping the back rounded
- ✓ Do not hold your breath. Breathe in and out throughout the exercise
- ✓ Use diaphragmatic breathing through the nose as much as possible
- ✓ Do not exercise to the point of strain or discomfort

## Side Bends  *Muscles worked: Obliques (Waist)*

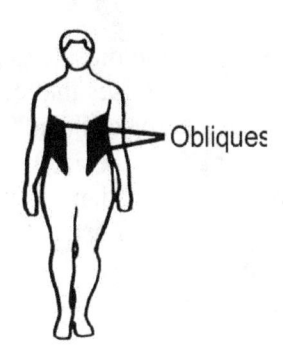

Obliques

Before starting, check your posture. Sit at the front edge of the chair as much as possible in order to engage your abdominal muscles. Inhale as you sit up straight.
Exhale and bend to the right as far as you can. Do not lean forward, keep the shoulders over the hips. The elbows stay straight. As you come back up, let the waist muscles lift you up, and do not lift the weight with the arm. Keep the shoulders down and relaxed. Do 8-12 repetitions on the right, then 8-12 repetitions on the left.

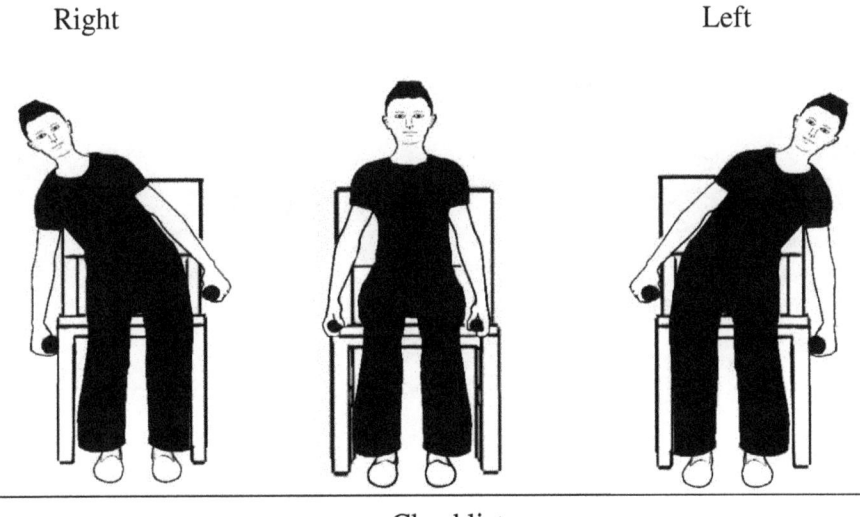

Right                                   Left

### Checklist
- ✓ Sit up straight, away from the back of the chair if possible
- ✓ Inhale as you sit up, exhale as you bend
- ✓ Keep the spine straight and the shoulders over the hips
- ✓ Do not bend the elbows or lift the weights when sitting up. The movement is all in the waist
- ✓ Move slowly using a "4 thousand count" both to bend to the side and to sit up straight
- ✓ Use diaphragmatic breathing through the nose as much as possible
- ✓ Do not exercise to the point of strain or discomfort

## Summary

There are many other exercises that work the same muscle groups, and many variations on the above exercises. There are also strengthening exercises that can be done using theraband, tubing, and physioballs, and your own body weight. The exercises listed in this chapter demonstrate a safe and complete workout and provide a good starting point. However, following the same exercise routine for long periods will eventually cause your body to adapt to the exercises, and you will discontinue getting good results. It is important to vary your exercise routine from time to time, trying different exercises and different forms of resistance.

After you become familiar with the various muscles you are trying to isolate and you become comfortable using resistance, try looking into other books, videos or classes to help vary your routine. When following any exercise program, remember to use good body mechanics and good form in order to protect your back and joints from injury.

*Remember, resistance exercises should always be done slowly and with control.*

# Chapter 5
## Yoga and Tai Chi For Flexibility and Balance

*"Courage doesn't always roar. Sometimes courage is the little
voice at the end of the day that says I'll try again tomorrow."*
- Mary Anne Radmacher

Balance problems are common in those with osteoporosis and they can increase the risk of a fall.
- Each year, about one-third of individuals 65 years of age or older will fall.
- Ten percent will fracture a bone, dislocate a joint, or incur some other serious injury.
- Nearly one-half of those who incur a serious injury never fully recover, and many lose their ability to function independently for the rest of their lives. A good proportion end up in nursing homes, making falls and the injuries that result one of the most substantial health threats facing older Americans.
- Each year approximately 9,500 fall-related deaths occur in older Americans.
- Various surveys show that 40 to 73 percent of people over age 60 who have fallen fear falling again, and half of those people restrict their activities as a result.

## *Causes of Falls*

Falls often occur due to medications such as sedatives, muscle relaxants, and blood pressure drugs, which can cause dizziness, lightheadedness, or loss of balance. When two or more medications are used in combination, these side effects may be aggravated. Other causes include diminished vision, hearing, muscle strength, coordination, and reflexes. Certain diseases can also affect balance. Falls often occur at home and are common when getting in and out of a chair or shower, stepping backwards, and reaching out too far to grab onto something. Many elderly people have a fear of falling, so they restrict their activities, beginning a downward spiral. Instead of becoming less active, they should be encouraged to do exercises that improve balance, strength, and help to maintain function thereby reducing the risk of falling.

Good balance is important to help you get around, remain independent, and carry out daily activities. Having good balance means being able to control and maintain your body's position whether you are moving or remaining still. An intact sense of balance helps you walk without staggering, rise from a chair without falling, and climb stairs more easily.

## *How Your Body Maintains Balance*

The body maintains balance by coordinating information received from three systems – vestibular (hearing), visual, and proprioceptive. The vestibular system works with the visual system to keep objects in focus when the head is moving. The proprioceptive system is comprised of joint and muscle receptors throughout the body that send signals to the brain to aid in maintaining balance. The brain receives, interprets, and processes the information from all of these systems in order to control balance.

### The Role of the Vestibular or Auditory System

This system helps maintain balance by sensing the movement and position of the head, and acceleration and deceleration of the body. This occurs through the semicircular canals which are three tiny, fluid-filled tubes in your inner ear. Movement of fluid in the semicircular canals signals the brain about the direction, speed, and rotation of the head, such as when nodding up and down or looking from right to left. When the head moves, the liquid inside the semicircular canals also moves. This in turn puts pressure on the tiny hairs that line each canal. These hairs translate the movement of the liquid into nerve messages that are sent to your brain. Your brain then can tell your body how to stay balanced.

### The Role of the Visual System

This system sends visual signals to the brain about the body's position in relation to its surroundings. These signals are processed by the brain, and compared to information from the vestibular and the proprioceptive systems. The visual system provides the brain with visual cues which are utilized as reference points in orienting the body in space.

### The Role of the Proprioceptive System

This system provides an information link between your brain and the more than 650 muscles that move your body. This system relies on feedback from skin pressure and muscle and joint sensory receptors to tell the brain what part of the body is touching the ground and what parts of the body are moving. This system is made up of receptor cells found within each muscle fiber and nerves that travel from the muscles through the spinal cord to the brain. This system utilizes specific communication patterns within the brain that interprets these signals, allowing your body to meet the ever-changing demands of movement and balance. When this system is functioning efficiently an individual's body position is automatically adjusted in different situations. The proprioceptive system is responsible for providing the body with the necessary signals to allow you to plan and execute different motor tasks such as sitting properly in a chair and stepping off a curb smoothly. It also allows the body to coordinate fine motor movements such as writing with a pencil, using a spoon to drink soup, and buttoning one's shirt. In order for this system to work properly, it must rely on obtaining accurate information from the sensory systems and then organizing and interpreting this information efficiently and effectively. Acting together, these three systems constantly gather and interpret sensory information from all over the body. This allows the body to act on that information in an appropriate and helpful way. The information from these systems travels to the central balance mechanism in your brain. In turn, the brain sends out signals allowing you to control your body movements, maintain your balance, and give you a sense of stability.

With age there are natural changes that occur that can affect balance. The fluid inside the ears can begin to dry out and the hairs can become less sensitive. Vision also often diminishes with age and the sensory receptors in the body lose some of their sensitivity. All of the above reduces the information that reaches the brain which can result in a diminished ability to maintain balance. Unfortunately these types of changes can not be avoided. However, even with these changes falls are not considered a normal part of aging and there are steps that can be taken to improve balance at any age. This includes being mindful about body mechanics as discussed in chapter one and keeping the body strong and flexible. A strong and flexible body can better adapt to movement and make the necessary corrections to keep the body balanced.

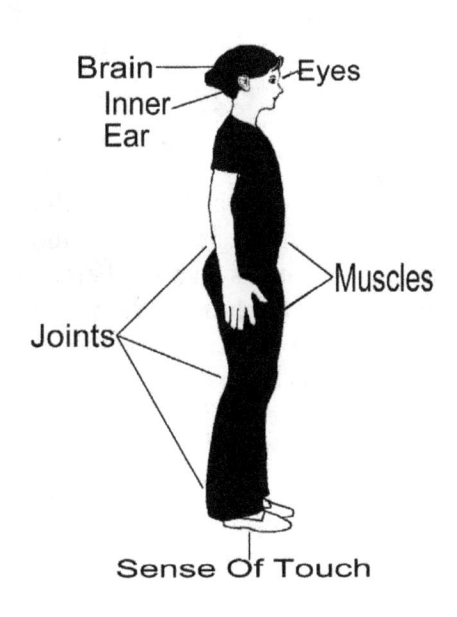

# How Yoga and Tai Chi Can Help Improve Your Balance

Age-related falls are caused in part by a reduced sense of balance and a loss of ability to judge body placement. Aging causes many changes in the body that can increase the chances of a fall. One change is a loss of hearing and less sensitivity in the auditory system. Changes in vision will lessen the information that the brain receives in order to keep the body straight. A loss of sensitivity in the proprioceptors can also occur. As the sensitivity of these systems diminishes the brain is left with less of the sensory information it needs to maintain balance. Slower reflexes, decreased muscle strength, loss of eyesight and depth perception all contribute to a diminished sense of equilibrium.

Changes in balance can also be the result of a sedentary lifestyle. Failure to exercise regularly results in poor muscle tone, decreased strength, and loss of bone mass and flexibility. All of these changes not only increase the likelihood of a fall but can also have an impact on the severity of any injury that might occur as a result of a fall.

Maintaining balance requires stability of the core muscles and the joints, particularly the hip, knee, and ankle. With age these areas often decline in muscle strength and size. Performing balance exercises challenges the nervous and muscular systems.

## *Flexibility and Range of Motion*

Flexibility refers to the ability to move the joints and muscles through their full range of motion. As you become more flexible and gain greater range of motion, you will find it easier to perform everyday activities such as reaching items on high shelves, looking behind you to back up the car or tying your shoes. The less you have to struggle to perform these activities, the less likely you are to fall and be injured. A regular stretching routine will lead to increased range of motion in the joints, better posture, protection against muscle injuries such as strains or sprains, improved circulation, and a reduction in muscle tension.

*Tips for Safe Stretching*

> - Stretch only to the point where you feel a gentle pull.
> - Do not stretch to the point of pain.
> - *Do not bounce while you stretch.* Bouncing can cause small tears in the muscle fibers creating less flexibility
> - Do not hold your breath while you stretch. Breathe evenly in-and-out during each stretch.
> - Hold each stretch approximately twenty to thirty seconds

One benefit of stretching is that it increases the length of both your muscles and tendons, leading to an increase in range of movement. A flexible joint has the ability to move through a greater range of motion while requiring less energy to do so. Daily stretching improves muscular balance and posture. Stretching also increases joint synovial fluid, which is a lubricating fluid that promotes the transport of more nutrients to the joints' articular cartilage. This allows a greater range of motion and can reduce joint degeneration. Improved muscle coordination is another benefit of regular stretching.

## The Benefits of a Yoga Practice

There are many misconceptions about what a yoga practice entails. The thought of yoga often conjures up images of having to sit cross legged on the floor for long periods, standing on one's head, chanting, being connected with a particular religion or spiritual belief, or wrapping oneself into a posture which seems impossible for the average human to do. Yoga is not about achieving advanced postures, sitting still for long periods, or being connected to a specific religious practice. The word yoga, taken from the Sanskrit word *"Yuj,"* simply means union; union of mind, body and spirit or soul, nothing more. The goal of yoga is to become more connected with your body and mind through the use of movement, breathwork and meditation or directed concentration.

The practice of yoga can help improve balance, increase flexibility, reduce stress, lower blood pressure, and aids in lessening common aches and pains. Yoga can be especially beneficial for those with injuries or chronic illness. Since yoga is about union of mind, body, and spirit, the main goal for the yoga student is to find the expression of the posture that best suits his or her individual and unique needs. It is about both a willingness to go inside to discover the movements that are best, and a willingness to honor those discoveries. Many traditional yoga postures can be adapted to accommodate all abilities, levels and ages. There are chair yoga classes in which every movement is performed sitting in a chair, and there are also programs for those who are bedridden. Yoga does not require one to follow any specific belief system to participate. The philosophies of yoga are universal and can be incorporated within any belief system. The warm up exercises introduced in chapter two are common movements used in yoga. Yoga can be a wonderful form of exercise, due to its slow and gentle nature. Many of the postures help improve balance and reduce the risk of falls. As the student of yoga gently and with respect for the body begins to increase flexibility, aches and pains in the back, knees, and hips may lessen as the muscles are stretched and the pressure exerted on the joints is reduced. Also, as flexibility increases, many of the activities of daily life become easier. When the muscles of the neck loosen it becomes easier to turn the head when trying to back up the car. When the muscles of the legs and back become more limber it becomes easier to reach or pick up items at varying heights. With an increased range of motion in the shoulder muscles, grooming and dressing tasks can become easier. As mentioned earlier the easier your everyday tasks become the less likely you are to fall.

Some of the benefits of a yoga practice include:
- Increased feelings of relaxation. Gentle stretching, breathing, meditation and guided relaxation releases body tension and calms the nervous system and emotions.
- Improved balance. Better focus, attention, and concentration are promoted through a yoga practice of mindful movement and enhanced body awareness. As you gain more body awareness you will be better able to judge when you are out of balance and can make corrections to prevent a fall. Muscles become more toned as they work to hold the yoga postures.
- Improved flexibility. Yoga gently stretches the muscles in the body increasing the flexibility and length of the muscles, tendons and ligaments.
- Improved energy levels. The slow, gentle movements combined with deep breathing help to energize the body.
- Lung capacity can improve. Yoga emphasizes deep diaphragmatic breathing that can help to strengthen the lungs and improve respiratory health.

## Yoga Breathing

An important component of yoga is the combination of deep breathing and movement. Through breathwork you will learn to release tension in the body and stretch to the appropriate level. This breathing is the same breath introduced in Chapter two and you should be familiar with this technique as it is the same breathing you have been using with all of the exercises in this book.

# The Poses

*Before beginning this sequence of yoga postures it is important to warm up the body.* Performing the yoga-based warm-up exercises in chapter two would be a good predecessor to the following movements. For all of the following postures *remember*, that yoga is about honoring the body's needs. With each posture, experiment to find a level of intensity where you are challenging yourself but not struggling. If the breathing becomes restricted or the only thought you have is how soon you can release the posture, you are pushing yourself too hard. If you find the above happening, lessen the stretch or come out of the posture sooner.

As with many of the movements in this book, the yoga postures will be shown standing, standing while holding on, and seated. Try to do as many postures as you can standing without holding on to help improve your balance.

## Concerns for those with osteoporosis

As beneficial as yoga is for osteoporosis precautions need to be taken. The first step is to speak with your doctor to find out if you have compression fractures and where they are located. You should also be aware of what your bone density test results are.

If you have severe osteoporosis or compression fractures you want to avoid twisting motions or rounding of the back. Both can cause compression fractures or make them worse. If you have either seek advise from a physician or physical therapist about how to proceed.

An important component of yoga is the combination of deep breathing and movement. The breath we will use with all of the postures is the same breath used throughout this book.

## Belly Breathing Seated

Sit up straight. Rest your hands across your abdomen. As you exhale through the nose, gently contract your abdominal muscles and push all of the air out of your belly and lungs.

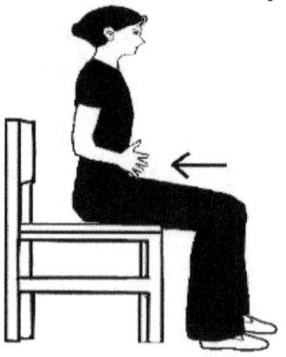

As you inhale through the nose let the belly rise first. Your belly and hands should move out with the inhalation. Then let the chest rise next. It may take some practice to have the belly move first. Do not let the shoulders rise up when inhaling. The shoulders stay down and relaxed the entire time.

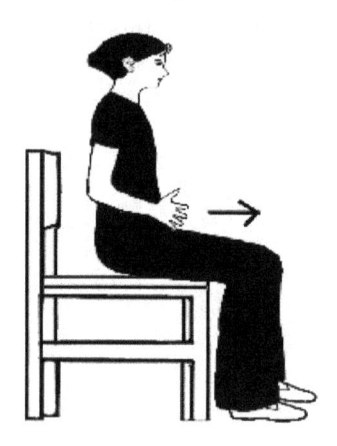

# Belly Breathing Lying Down

Lie on your back on the floor. Rest your hands across your abdomen.
As you exhale through the nose, gently contract your abdominal muscles and push all of the air out of your belly and lungs.

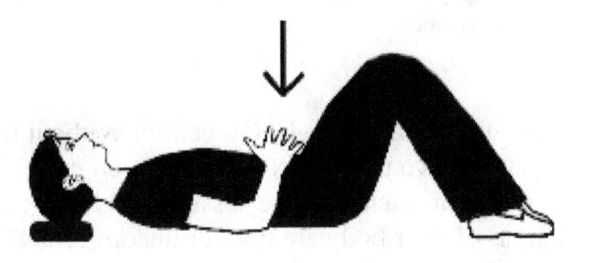

   As you inhale through the nose let the belly rise first. Your belly and hands should move out with the inhalation. Then let the chest rise next. It may take some practice to have the belly move first. To help learn how to move the belly correctly, you can place a pillow on the stomach and try to make it rise and fall with the breath.

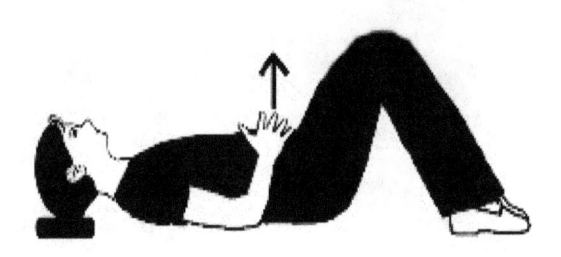

# Warm Up

For all of the following postures remember, that yoga is about honoring the body's needs. With each posture experiment to find a level of intensity where you are challenging yourself but not struggling. If the breathing becomes restricted or the only thought you have is how soon you can release the posture, you are pushing yourself too hard. If you find the above happening, lessen the stretch or come out of the posture sooner.

The following movements should be done slowly and gently. Without forcing, try to increase your range of motion with each repetition. Do not push your body to do more than feels right. Since each day with osteoporosis can be different, each exercise session will be as well. Use this segment as an opportunity to notice which areas of your body are tight or uncomfortable, and which areas move more easily. This process will help you to determine which postures are appropriate to do, and how vigorous or gently you should proceed with the standing and/or floor work.

## Half Neck Rolls

If possible sit at the front edge of the chair allowing your abdominal muscles to hold you up straight. If you are experiencing discomfort or find yourself slouching, slide all the way back in the chair so your back remains straight.

Drop your right ear to your right shoulder and then make a half circle by rolling your chin to your chest and then rolling the left ear to the left shoulder. Reverse the movement making a half circle from left to right. It is not recommended to drop the head backwards as this compresses the neck. Exhale as you circle your chin to your chest and inhale as you roll the ear to the shoulder. Use deep belly breathing through just the nose as much as possible.

Do this movement slowly and gently, counting *one-one thousand, two-one thousand, three-one thousand, four-one thousand* each time you circle your chin to your chest, and use the same count each time you roll the ear to the shoulder. Go for 8-12 repetitions. One repetition involves going to both sides.

Drop your right ear to your right shoulder.

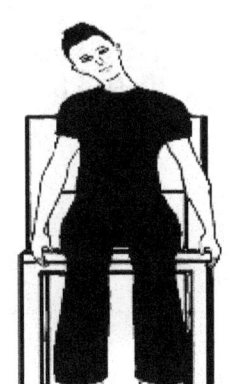

Circle your chin to your chest.

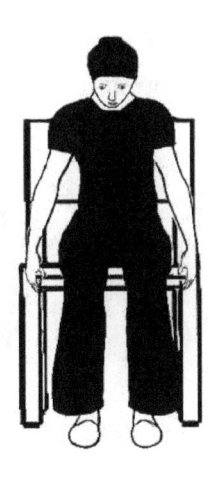

Circle your left ear to your left shoulder.

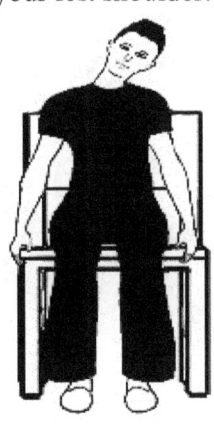

---

### Checklist
- ✓ Sit up straight
- ✓ Do not turn the head, look straight forward
- ✓ Move slowly using a "4 thousand count" for each movement
- ✓ Exhale as you circle the chin to the chest, and inhale as you roll the ear to the shoulder
- ✓ Use diaphragmatic breathing through the nose as much as possible
- ✓ Do not exercise to the point of strain or discomfort

## Neck Stretch

After circling 8-12 times, hold to the right, press the right ear to the right shoulder. Do not turn your head or chin, look straight forward to stretch the side of the neck. Each time you exhale let the right ear drop closer to the right shoulder and gently press the left shoulder down a bit more. Hold for 5-10 deep belly breaths. Then hold to the left.

Hold Right                                  Hold Left

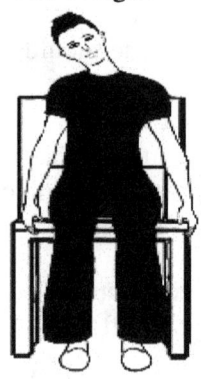

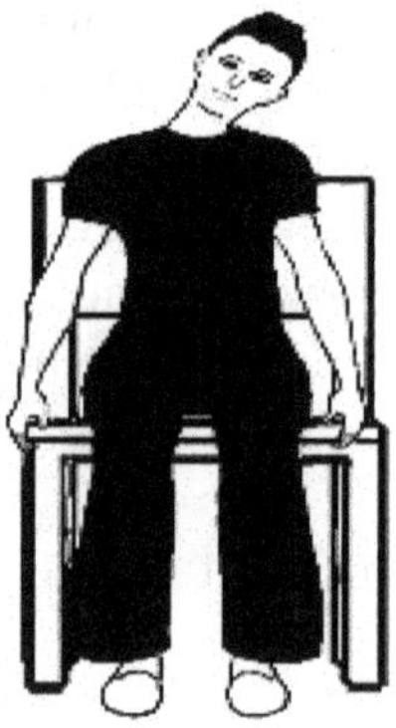

Next, drop the chin to the chest, and hold. Sit up straight. With each exhale roll the shoulders back and down and gently drop the chin, stretching the back of the neck. Hold for 5-10 deep belly breaths.

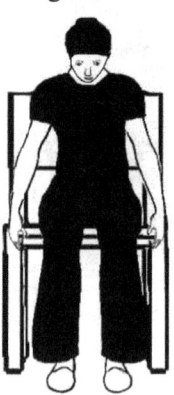

### Checklist
- ✓ Sit up straight
- ✓ Do not turn the head, look straight forward
- ✓ Do this stretch once in each direction
- ✓ Hold each stretch for 5-10 deep belly breaths
- ✓ Use diaphragmatic breathing through the nose as much as possible
- ✓ Do not exercise to the point of strain or discomfort

## Head Rotation

Bring the head back to a neutral position. Check to see that you are still sitting up straight and away from the back of the chair if possible.

Keeping your chin parallel to the floor, turn your head to the right to look over the right shoulder. Come back to center. Then turn the head to the left and look over the left shoulder. Come back to center. Exhale each time you turn the head to the side. Inhale each time you come back to center. Do this movement slowly and gently, counting *one-one thousand, two-one thousand, three-one thousand, four-one thousand* each time you turn to the side. Use the same count as you come back to the center, and again each time you turn the head to the other side. Do this movement 8-12 times. One repetition involves going to both sides.

Turning the head to the right.   Turning the head to the left.

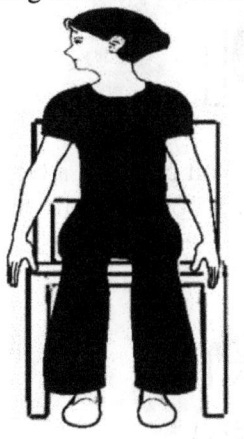

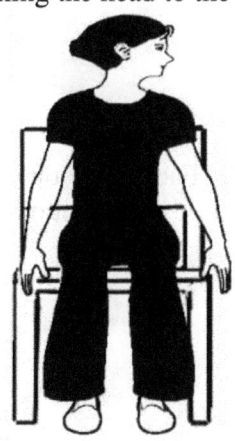

### Checklist
- ✓ Sit up straight
- ✓ Move slowly using a "4 thousand count" for each movement
- ✓ Use diaphragmatic breathing through the nose as much as possible
- ✓ Do not exercise to the point of strain or discomfort

## Head Rotation Stretch

After completing 8-12 repetitions. Hold to the right side looking over the right shoulder. Each time you exhale see if you can look a bit more to the right and gently press the left shoulder back a bit more. Hold for 5-10 deep belly breaths.

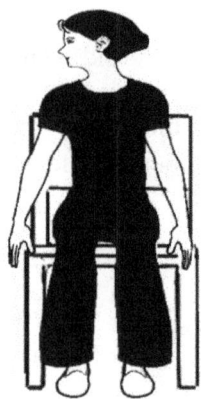

Then hold to the left side. Each time you exhale see if you can look a bit more to the left and gently press the right shoulder back a bit more. Hold for 5-10 deep belly breaths.

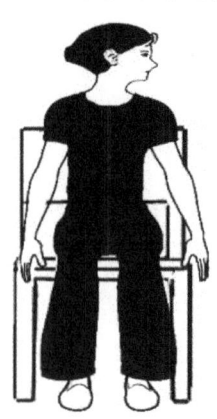

| Checklist |
|---|
| ✓ Sit up straight |
| ✓ Do the stretches once in each direction |
| ✓ Hold each stretch for 5-10 deep belly breaths |
| ✓ Use diaphragmatic breathing through the nose as much as possible |
| ✓ Do not exercise to the point of strain or discomfort |

## Chin Tuck

This movement should be done gently just a few times. This exercise helps to strengthen the muscles in the back of the neck. This will help to correct the forward head position common in those with osteoporosis.

Bring the head to a neutral position. Check to see if you are still sitting up straight and away from the back of the chair if possible. Keeping the chin parallel to the floor, gently retract or draw the chin back straightening the back of the neck. Exhale as you draw the head back and inhale as you release forward. Do this movement slowly and gently, counting *one-one thousand, two-one thousand, three-one thousand, four-one thousand* each time you draw the chin back. Use the same count as you release the chin forward.

Neutral positionDraw the chin straight back

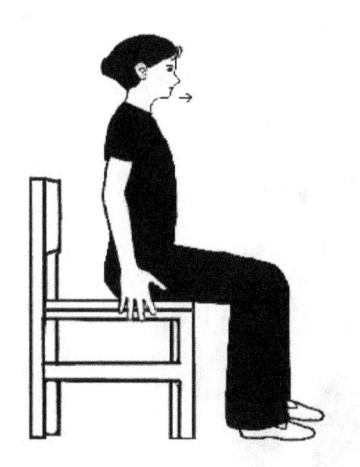

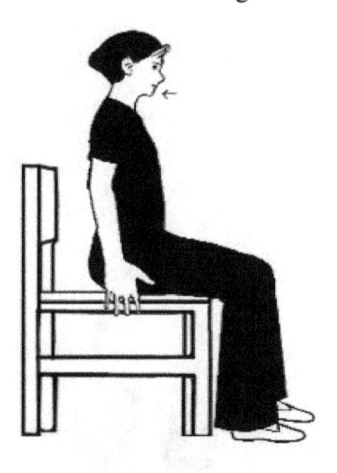

| Checklist |
|---|
| ✓ Sit up straight |
| ✓ Move slowly using a "4 thousand count" for each movement |
| ✓ Keep the chin parallel to the floor |
| ✓ Use diaphragmatic breathing through the nose as much as possible |
| ✓ Do not exercise to the point of strain or discomfort |

## Shoulder Rolls

Bring the head back to a neutral position. Check to see if you are still sitting up straight and away from the back of the chair if possible.

Lift the shoulders up towards the ears as high as you can in a shrugging motion. Then roll the shoulders down and back, pressing them down as far as you can. Do this movement slowly and gently, counting *one-one thousand, two-one thousand, three-one thousand, four-one thousand* each time you lift the shoulders. Use the same count as you lower the shoulders. Repeat for 8-12 shoulder rolls. Inhale as you lift the shoulders up and exhale as you press the shoulders down. Exaggerate at both ends of the movement. Make sure you do not bend the elbows. The arms stay straight and the movement is all in the shoulders. This is an area which can become stiff, so it is helpful to look in a mirror or have someone watch you do this movement to make sure the shoulders are both lifting up and pressing down.

Press the shoulders down      Roll the shoulders up

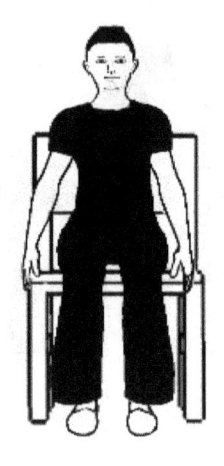

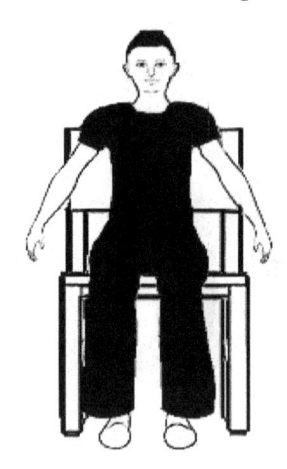

### Checklist
- ✓ Sit up straight
- ✓ Use diaphragmatic breathing through the nose as much as possible
- ✓ Move slowly using a "4 thousand count" for each movement
- ✓ Make sure you are lifting the shoulders up and lowering them down
- ✓ Do not bend the elbows, keep the arms straight
- ✓ Do not exercise to the point of strain or discomfort

# Overhead Strap Stretch

These next two stretches are helpful for increasing the range of motion in the shoulder and correcting posture. You can do these stretches with a yoga strap or use a long sheet or towel.

Check to see if you are still sitting up straight. For this stretch sit up against the back of the chair. Hold the strap or towel in the hands with the palms facing down. The further apart the hands are the easier this stretch is. Inhale as you lift the strap up overhead. Then exhale as you bring the strap behind the head and back behind you as far as you possibly can. Then gently pull on the strap and bring it back to the starting position. Do not duck your head to bring the strap back around. If you need a gentler stretch bring your hand further apart. Do this movement slowly and gently, counting *one-one thousand, two-one thousand, three-one thousand, four-one thousand* each time you lift the strap back. Use the same count as you bring the strap forward.

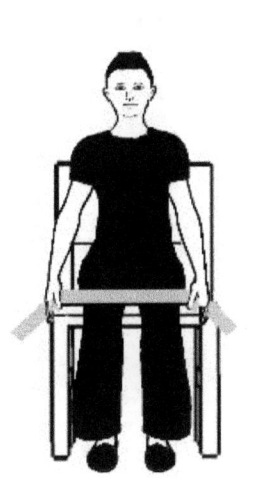

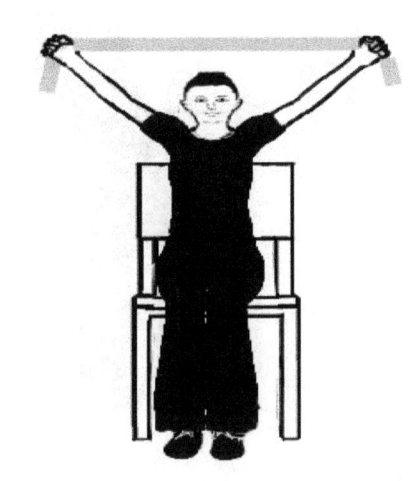

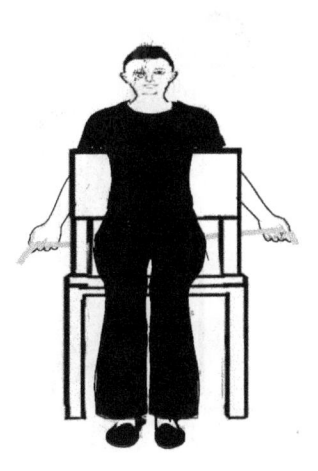

Checklist
- ✓ Sit up straight against the back of the chair
- ✓ Use diaphragmatic breathing through the nose as much as possible
- ✓ Move slowly using a "4 thousand count" for each movement
- ✓ Only bring the strap back behind you as far as you can without hurting the shoulders
- ✓ Do not bend the elbows, keep the arms straight
- ✓ Do not exercise to the point of strain or discomfort

## Side to Side Strap Stretch

Check to see if you are still sitting up straight. For this stretch sit up against the back of the chair. Hold the strap or towel in the hands with the palms facing down. The further apart the hands are the easier this stretch is. Inhale as you lift the strap up overhead. Then exhale as you bend to the right. Keep a gentle pull on the strap. If possible look up at the top hand. If that hurts the neck look straight ahead. Hold for 5 to 10 deep breaths and focus on drawing the arms and shoulders back. Release and repeat to the left.

Stretch to the right Stretch to the left

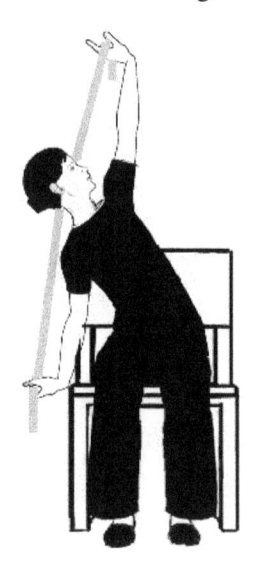

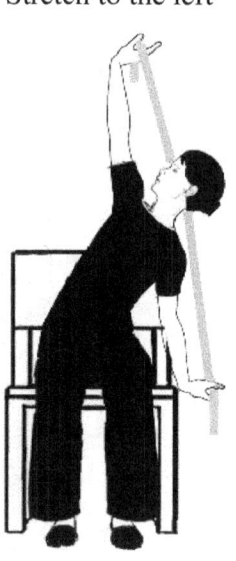

### Checklist
- ✓ Sit up straight against the back of the chair
- ✓ Use diaphragmatic breathing through the nose as much as possible
- ✓ Hold for 5 to 10 deep breaths in each direction
- ✓ Do not twist the body as you bend side to side.
- ✓ Do not bend the elbows, keep the arms straight
- ✓ Do not exercise to the point of strain or discomfort

## Seated Cat Stretch

This next stretch is designed to help loosen the low back muscles. The low back is an area that often becomes tight and prone to injury. This area is often neglected in many exercise routines and it is a difficult area to learn to isolate. This is another movement where it is helpful to have someone watch to see if you are performing the movement correctly. A common mistake is to just lean back with the whole body instead of rounding the low back. In order to correctly loosen these muscles it is important to learn to isolate the low back area during this movement.

Check that you are sitting up straight and away from the back of the chair. For this exercise, you need to be at the very front edge of the seat in order to move the low back. First push the abdomen forward and the shoulders back to create an arch in the low back. Do not drop the head back.

Next, let the shoulders round forward, pull the abdominal muscles in, and let the low back round out. Think of a cat arching its back. Again, it is your low back, not the upper back or shoulders, that is moving closer to the back of the chair.

Go back and forth between arching the low back and rounding the low back. Inhale as you arch the back and exhale as you round the back. Do this movement slowly and gently, counting *one-one thousand, two-one thousand, three-one thousand, four-one thousand* as you round back and use the same count each time you arch the back. Do this movement 8-12 times. One repetition involves going both forward and back.

Arch the back                      Round the back

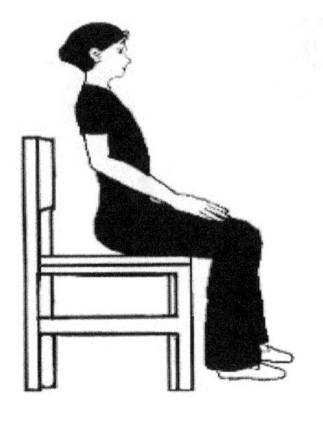

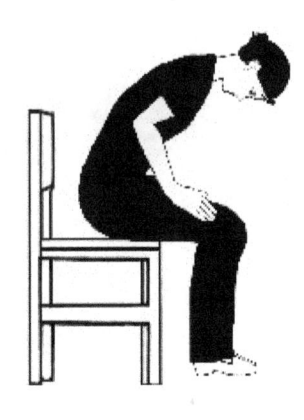

### Checklist
- ✓ Sit up straight
- ✓ Move slowly using a "4 thousand count" for each movement
- ✓ Use diaphragmatic breathing through the nose as much as possible
- ✓ Make sure you are isolating and rounding the low back and not just leaning back with the whole body
- ✓ Do not exercise to the point of strain or discomfort

## Chest Opener

This movement is helpful to stretch the shoulders and open the chest. If you have any sensitivities in your shoulders do this movement gently until you know how it will affect your shoulders.

Check that you are sitting up straight and away from the back of the chair if possible. Clasp your hands behind your head or neck. Do not pull the head forward. Use the chin tuck exercise (pg. 135) to keep your neck in alignment. If you can not bring your hands together behind your neck, you can bring your fingertips to the sides of your head. As you continue these stretches, you may find that your flexibility increases. Next, bring the elbows to the front as close together as you can. Again, do not pull the head forward; just go as far as you can with good alignment.

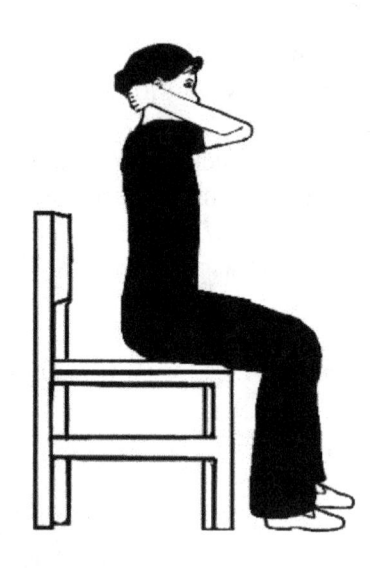

Next, open the shoulders up, bringing the elbows back as far as you comfortably can. Let the chest come forward and the low back arch slightly. Gently press the back of the head into the hands and squeeze the shoulder blades together in the back. Keep the shoulders down away from the ears.

Inhale as you open the elbows, and exhale as the elbows come together. Do this movement slowly and gently, *counting one-one thousand, two-one thousand, three-one thousand, four-one thousand* each time you open the elbows and use the same count each time you bring the elbows together. Do this movement 8-12 times. One repetition involves going both ways. Try to take deep breaths as you bring the elbows back. This movement opens the chest allowing the lungs to fully expand.

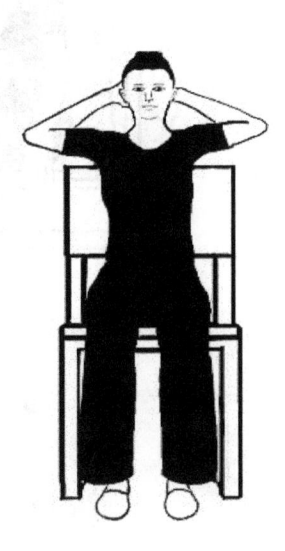

| Checklist |
|---|
| ✓ Sit up straight |
| ✓ Move slowly using a "4 thousand count" for each movement |
| ✓ Use diaphragmatic breathing through the nose as much as possible |
| ✓ Do not pull your head forward with your hands |
| ✓ Do not exercise to the point of strain or discomfort |

Before proceeding to standing movements, it is good to warm up the feet and ankles. These movements are helpful if you have been sitting for some time. Many falls happen while transitioning from sitting to standing. Sitting for long periods can reduce the circulation in the legs, impairing balance. These next two movements will help to restore circulation to the legs.

### Toe Lifts

Check that you are sitting up straight and away from the back of the chair if possible. Keeping the heels on the floor, lift both toes off the floor as high as you can. Repeat 8-12 times.

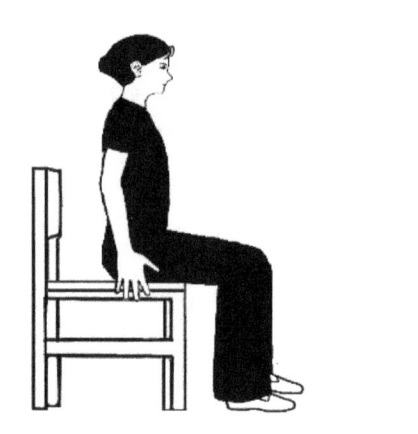

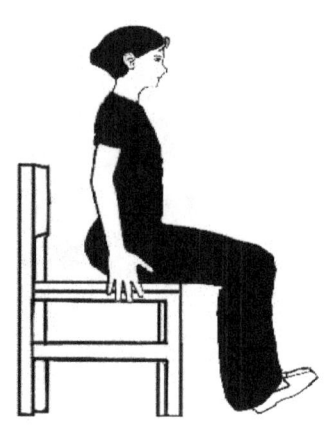

Checklist
- ✓ Sit up straight
- ✓ Move slowly using a "4 thousand count" for each movement
- ✓ Use diaphragmatic breathing through the nose as much as possible
- ✓ Do not exercise to the point of strain or discomfort

# Heel Lifts

Check that you are sitting up straight and away from the back of the chair if possible. Keeping the toes on the floor, lift both heels off the floor as high as you can. Repeat 8-12 times.
You can also alternate between these two movements i.e., lift the toes and then the heels, and continue back and forth.

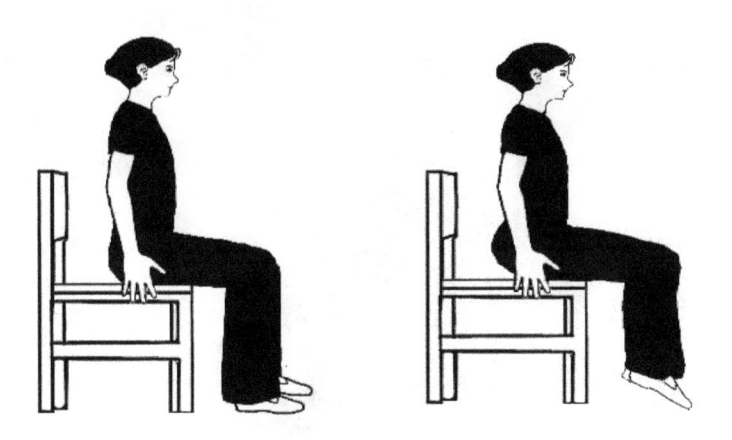

---

### Checklist
- ✓ Sit up straight
- ✓ Move slowly using a "4 thousand count" for each movement
- ✓ Use diaphragmatic breathing through the nose as much as possible
- ✓ Do not exercise to the point of strain or discomfort

## Ankle Circles

Check that you are sitting up straight and away from the back of the chair if possible. Lift the right foot off the floor and circle it clockwise and counter clockwise 8-12 times in each direction. Then switch to the left foot.

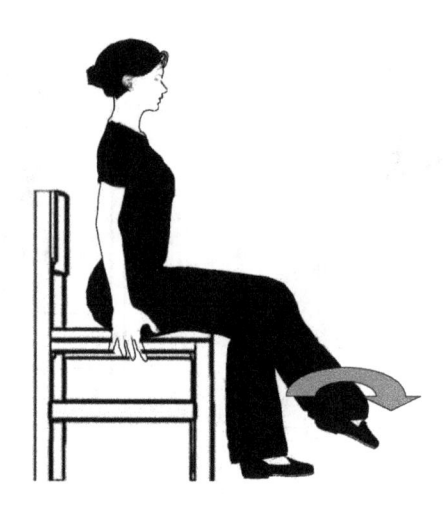

| Checklist |
|---|
| ✓ Sit up straight |
| ✓ Move slowly using a "4 thousand count" for each movement |
| ✓ Use diaphragmatic breathing through the nose as much as possible |
| ✓ Do not exercise to the point of strain or discomfort |

## Mountain Pose

Check your posture before you begin. Shoulders should be back and down and over the hips. Knees should remain slightly bent. Tuck in the chin and think about pushing the crown of the head up to the ceiling without lifting your chin. The abdominal muscles are lightly pulled in, but not so much that it restricts your breathing.

Stand up straight and lift your arms up overhead with the palms facing each other. Bring the arms back so the elbows are in line with the ears if possible. Drop the shoulders and line them up over the hips. Keep the knees slightly bent and the natural curve in the low back. Toes point straight forward. Place equal weight on both feet. Check that there is equal weight on the outside and inside of the foot, and on all of the toes so you are not rolling your ankles in or out. Check that there is equal weight on the ball and heel of the foot so you are not leaning forward or back. Hold for 5-10 deep belly breaths, or to comfort.

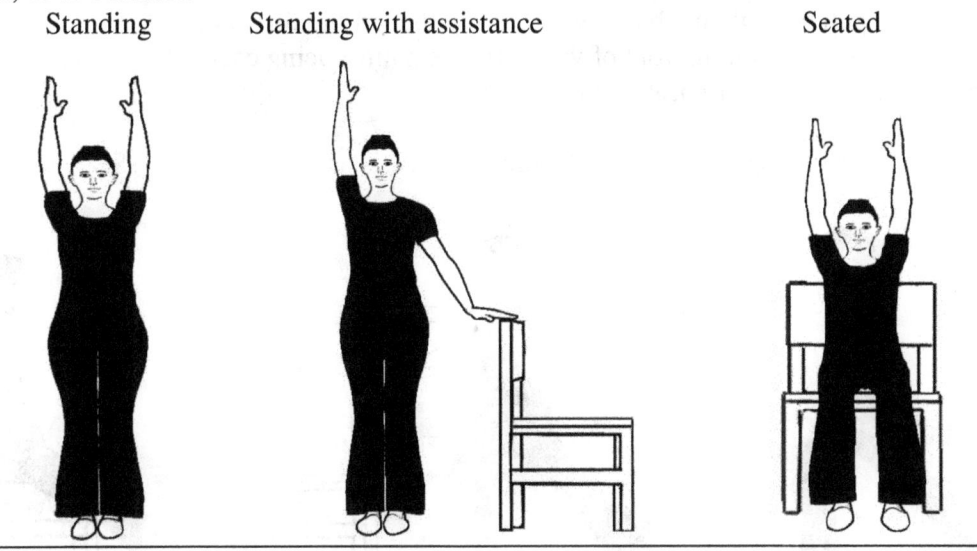

Standing     Standing with assistance     Seated

### Checklist
- ✓ Stand or sit up straight, away from the back of the chair if possible
- ✓ Keep the spine straight and the shoulders over the hips
- ✓ Keep the shoulders down away from the ears
- ✓ Keep the knees slightly bent and the natural curve in the low back
- ✓ Hold for 5-10 deep belly breaths, or to comfort
- ✓ Use diaphragmatic breathing through the nose as much as possible
- ✓ Do not exercise to the point of strain or discomfort
- ✓ Remember the goal of yoga is to find that point where you are challenging yourself but not struggling

## Warrior I Pose

Check your posture before you begin. Shoulders should be back and down and over the hips. Knees should remain slightly bent. Tuck in the chin and think about pushing the crown of the head up to the ceiling without lifting your chin. The abdominal muscles are lightly pulled in, but not so much that it restricts your breathing.

To start step your left leg back into a lunge position. Both feet should be pointing straight forward; do not turn your back foot or leg out to the side. Make sure that your right knee does not extend past your right ankle bone. You should be able to look down at your right knee and see both your right toes and the arch of the right foot. If you need a deeper stretch step the feet wider apart rather then lunging the right knee beyond the front toes. This will help to protect the knee joint from injury. Lift the back heel off of the floor. Bring the hips under the shoulders, do not lean the upper body forward. Gently pull the right hip back, as you bring the left hip forward. Without lifting the shoulders, reach the arms out in front of you, with the palms facing each other. Hold for 5-10 deep belly breaths, or to comfort. Repeat on the left side.

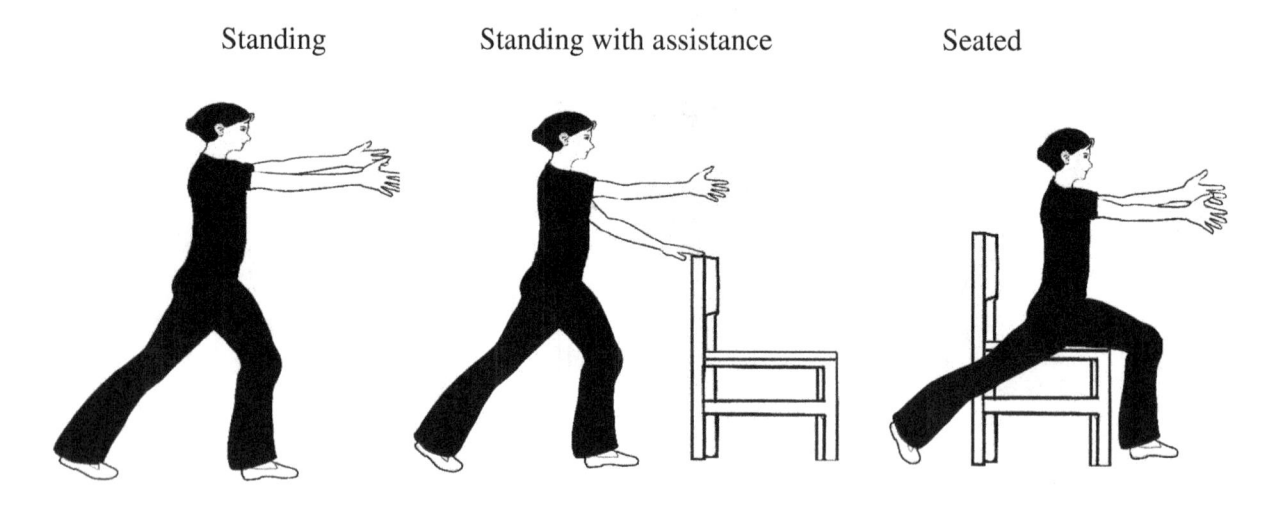

Standing     Standing with assistance     Seated

### Checklist
- ✓ Stand or sit up straight
- ✓ Keep the spine straight and the shoulders over the hips
- ✓ Keep the shoulders down away from the ears
- ✓ Keep the knees slightly bent and the natural curve in the low back
- ✓ Keep the front knee aligned over the front ankle
- ✓ Hold for 5-10 deep belly breaths, or to comfort
- ✓ Use diaphragmatic breathing through the nose as much as possible
- ✓ Do not exercise to the point of strain or discomfort
- ✓ Remember the goal of yoga is to find that point where you are challenging yourself but not struggling

## Warrior II Pose

Check your posture before you begin. Shoulders should be back and down and over the hips. Knees should remain slightly bent. Tuck in the chin and think about pushing the crown of the head up to the ceiling without lifting your chin. The abdominal muscles are lightly pulled in, but not so much that it restricts your breathing.

Step your right foot out to the side into a lunge position. The back knee is straight, but not locked and the front knee is bent. Turn the toes of the left foot in, so the left foot is at about a 45-degree angle. Turn the right toes out. Make sure that your right knee does not extend past your right ankle bone. You should be able to look down at your right knee and see both your right toes and the arch of the right foot. Also check that your right knee is directly over your ankle and not rolling in or out. If you need a deeper stretch step the feet wider apart rather then lunging the right knee forward beyond the toes. This will help to protect the knee joint from injury. Bring the arms out to the side about shoulder height with the palms facing the floor. Look out over your right hand. Bring the hips under the shoulders, do not lean the upper body forward. Hold for 5-10 deep belly breaths, or to comfort. Repeat on the left side.

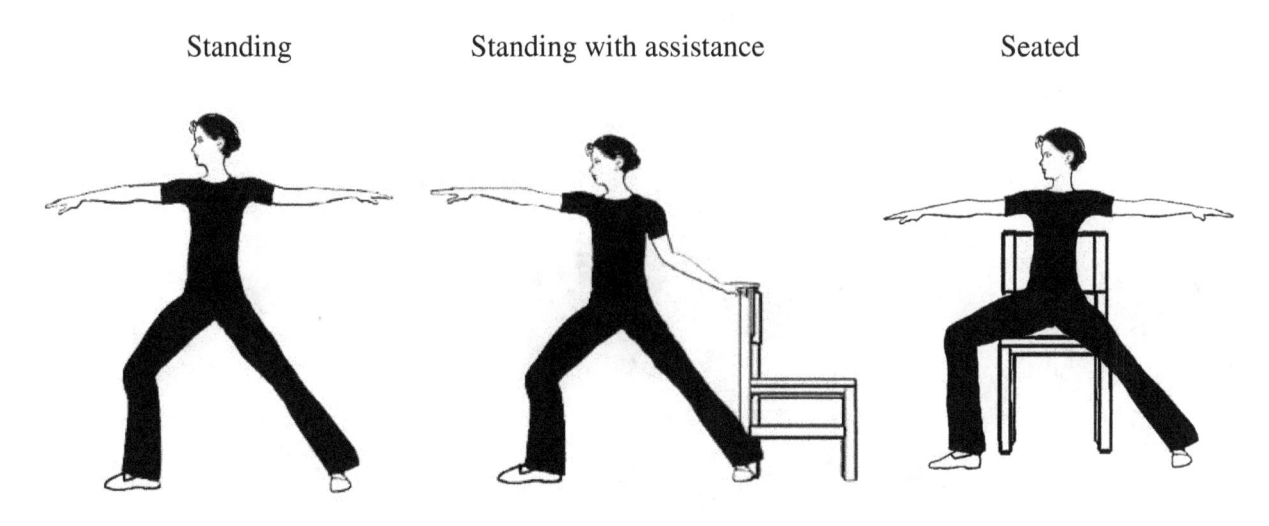

Standing        Standing with assistance        Seated

### Checklist
- ✓ Stand or sit up straight
- ✓ Keep the spine straight and the shoulders over the hips
- ✓ Keep the shoulders down away from the ears
- ✓ Keep the knees slightly bent and the natural curve in the low back
- ✓ Keep the bent knee aligned over the ankle
- ✓ Hold for 5-10 deep belly breaths, or to comfort
- ✓ Use diaphragmatic breathing through the nose as much as possible
- ✓ Do not exercise to the point of strain or discomfort
- ✓ Remember the goal of yoga is to find that point where you are challenging yourself but not struggling

## Lateral Angle Pose

If you have moderate to severe osteoporosis, a history of compression fractures, or if you have experienced a postural change or loss of height, check with your health care provider about the appropriateness of side bending exercises.

Check your posture before you begin. Shoulders should be back and down and over the hips. Knees should remain slightly bent. Tuck in the chin and think about pushing the crown of the head up to the ceiling without lifting your chin. The abdominal muscles are lightly pulled in, but not so much that it restricts your breathing. Step your right foot out to the side into a lunge position. The back knee is straight but not locked, and the front knee is bent. Turn the toes of the left foot in, so the foot is at about a 45-degree angle. Turn the right toes out. Make sure that your right knee does not extend past your right ankle bone. You should be able to look down at your right knee and see both your right toes and the arch of the right foot. Also check that your right knee is directly over your ankle and not rolling in or out. If you need a deeper stretch step the feet wider apart rather then lunging the right knee forward beyond the toes. Reach out to the right and bring your right hand (or for a deeper stretch your right elbow) to your right knee. Drop the left hip down making a straight line from your heel to your shoulder. Look up at your left hand if possible. If this is too strenuous just look straight ahead. Draw the left arm back to open the chest. *Do not lean the upper body forward.* Hold for 5-10 deep belly breaths, or to comfort. Repeat on the left side.

   Standing     Standing with assistance     Seated

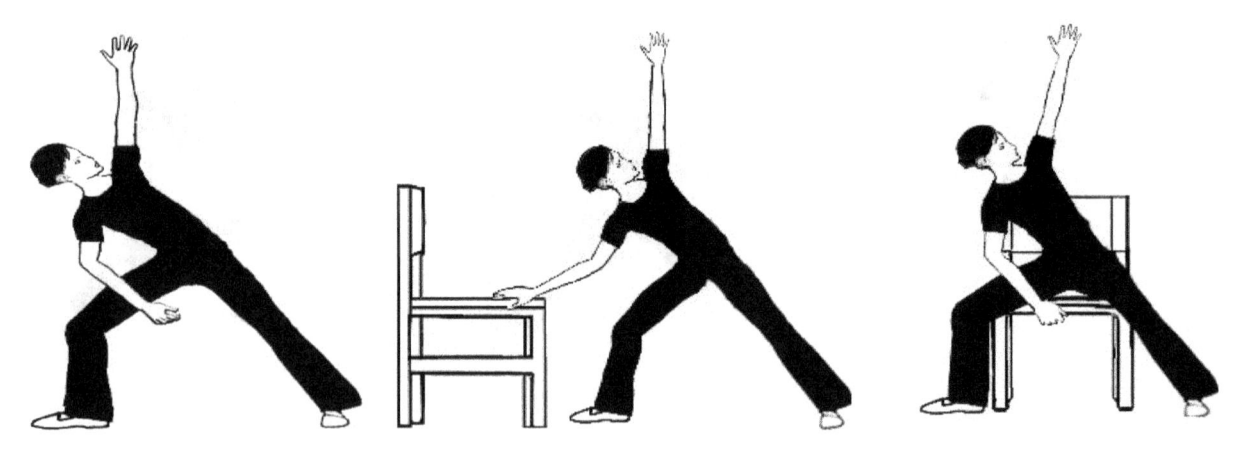

---

### Checklist
- ✓ Stand or sit up straight
- ✓ Keep the shoulders down away from the ears
- ✓ Keep the knees slightly bent and the natural curve in the low back
- ✓ Keep the front knee aligned over the front ankle
- ✓ Hold for 5-10 deep belly breaths, or to comfort
- ✓ Use diaphragmatic breathing through the nose as much as possible
- ✓ Do not exercise to the point of strain or discomfort
- ✓ Remember the goal of yoga is to find that point where you are challenging yourself but not struggling

## Standing Half Moon Pose

If you have moderate to severe osteoporosis, a history of compression fractures, or if you have experienced a postural change or loss of height, you should check with your healthcare provider about the appropriateness of side bending movements.

Clasp your hands overhead or hold onto the chair with one arm. Reach up and then side bend to the right. Do not lean forward, keep the shoulders over the hips. Do not let the top arm come forward, keep it over your head. Bring the elbows as close to the ears as you can. Each time you exhale see if you can bend a bit further to your right and bring the arms back closer to your ears.

*With this posture it is important to elongate the spine. Try to not just lean or bend to the side, but rather think about reaching up and lengthening through the ribcage and waist.* Each time you exhale see if you can reach up higher, bringing the arms closer to the ears and lengthening the waist. Hold for 5-10 deep belly breaths. Repeat on the left.

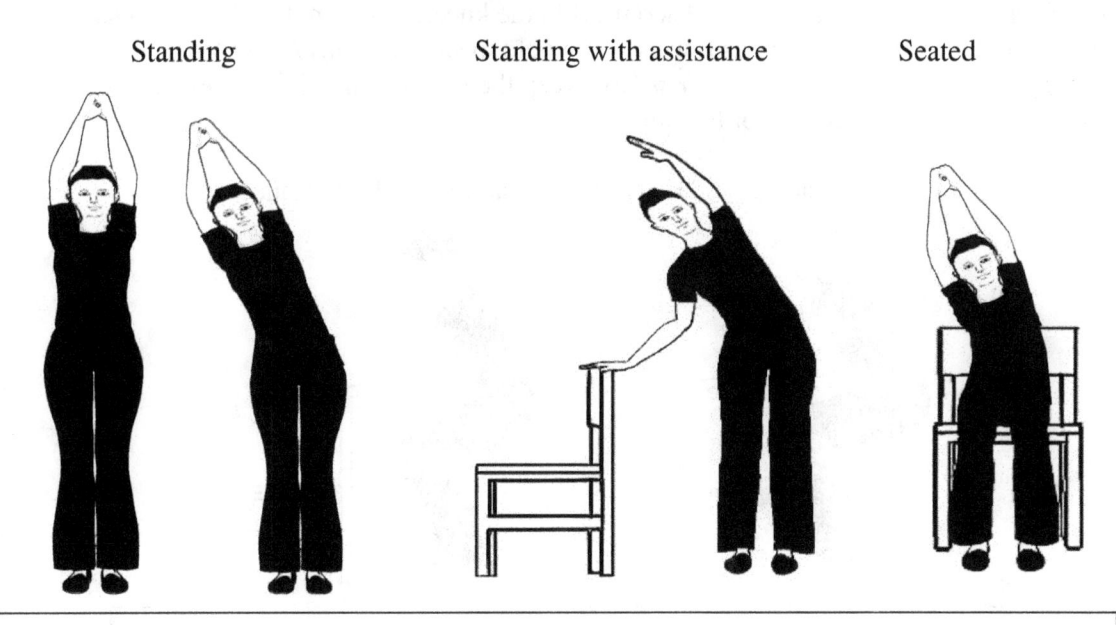

Standing        Standing with assistance        Seated

### Checklist
- ✓ Stand or sit up straight
- ✓ Do the stretches once in each direction
- ✓ Do not lean forward or let the top arm come forward. Keep the shoulders over the hips
- ✓ Hold each stretch for 5-10 deep belly breaths
- ✓ Use diaphragmatic breathing through the nose as much as possible
- ✓ Keep the knees slightly bent
- ✓ Do not exercise to the point of strain or discomfort

## Chair Pose

This posture is only shown standing, as there is no comparable seated version. If you are unable to do standing work, skip ahead to the next page.

Check your posture before you begin. Shoulders should be back and down and over the hips. Knees should remain slightly bent. Tuck in the chin and think about pushing the crown of the head up to the ceiling without lifting your chin. The abdominal muscles are lightly pulled in, but not so much that it restricts your breathing.

Without lifting the shoulders up, raise your arms out in front of you about shoulder height with the palms facing each other. Begin to bend the knees, reaching the buttocks back just as if you were about to sit in a chair. Keep your weight forward into the toes to avoid falling backwards. Make sure that your knees do not extend past your ankle bones. You should be able to look down at your knees and see both your toes and the arches of both feet. You should feel this posture in the thigh muscles, not the knee joints. The closer the feet are together, the more challenging this posture is. If you feel unsteady, step the feet wider apart. If you wish to challenge yourself more, bring the feet together. Go as low as you can without causing discomfort in the knees, but do not let the buttocks go below the knees. In other words, only go as low as you would to sit in a chair. *If you tend to fall backwards, place a chair behind you for safety.* Keep the natural curve in the low back.
Hold for 5-10 deep belly breaths, or to comfort.

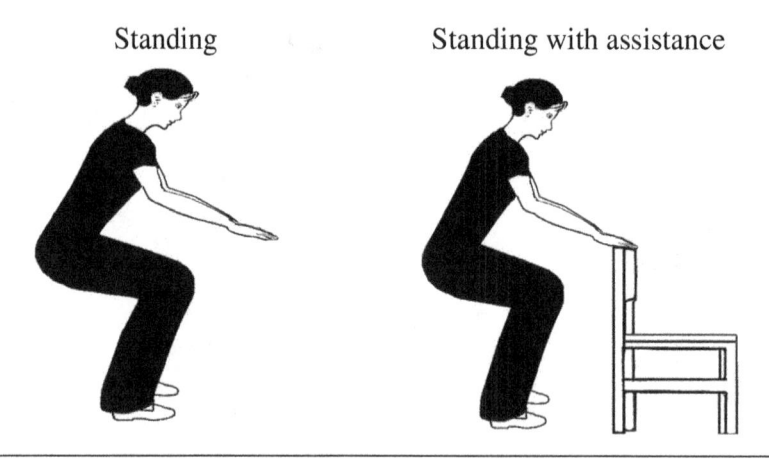

Standing      Standing with assistance

### Checklist
- ✓ Stand up straight
- ✓ Keep the shoulders down away from the ears
- ✓ Keep the knees slightly bent and the natural curve in the low back
- ✓ Keep the knees aligned over the ankles
- ✓ Hold for 5-10 deep belly breaths, or to comfort
- ✓ Use diaphragmatic breathing through the nose as much as possible
- ✓ Do not exercise to the point of strain or discomfort
- ✓ Remember the goal of yoga is to find that point where you are challenging yourself but not struggling

## Salutation To The Sun

If you have moderate to severe osteoporosis, a history of compression fractures, or if you have experienced a postural change or loss of height, check with your health care provider about the appropriateness of this exercise. The Salutation to the Sun is a series of postures that flow from one to the other. The challenge for those with or at risk for osteoporosis is performing this sequence while maintaining a straight and elongated spine. The following shows both the full version bringing the hand to the floor as well as a modification of the series utilizing a chair to help keep the back straight. The more challenging floor variation is geared to those without compression fractures.
If using a chair, place it up against a wall so when you lean on it the chair does not slide.

Check your posture before you begin. Shoulders should be back and down and over the hips. Knees should remain slightly bent. Tuck in the chin and think about pushing the crown of the head up to the ceiling without lifting your chin. The abdominal muscles are lightly pulled in, but not so much that it restricts your breathing.

Bring the palms together in prayer position in front of the heart. With the palms together raise the arms overhead. If it feels appropriate lengthen up from the waist and do a gentle back bend. If back bending does not feel right skip this movement. Make sure you do not drop the head back and compress the neck. Just look slightly up at an angle. Then come back up straight.

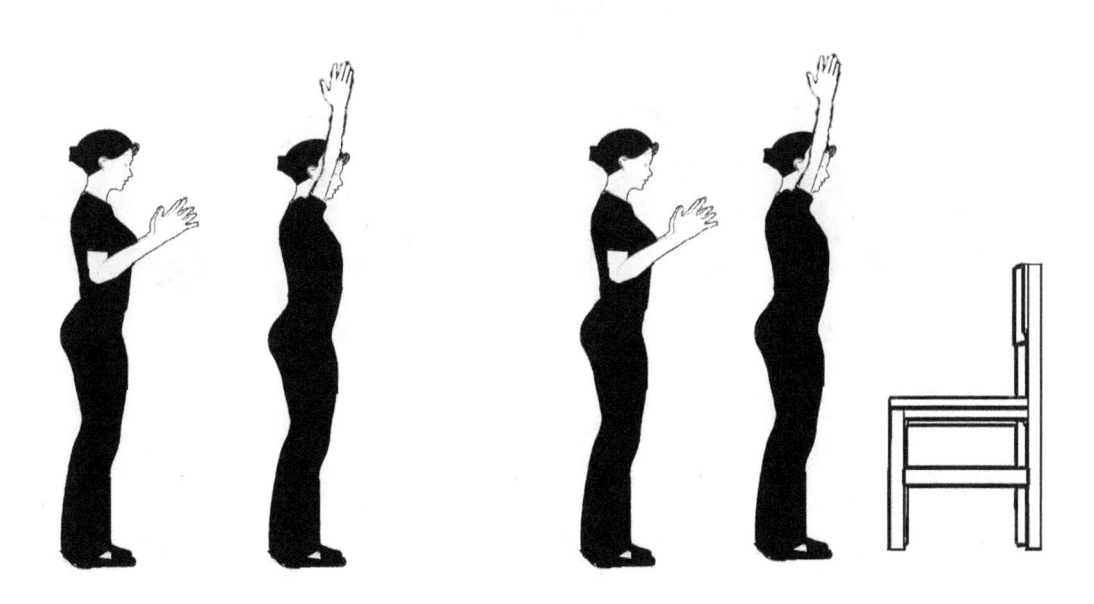

## Forward Bend

Bend your knees as much as you can. This will help to protect the back. Hip hinge or bend at the hips and come into forward bend keeping the back straight. Do not round the back. Bring your hands to the chair or the floor.

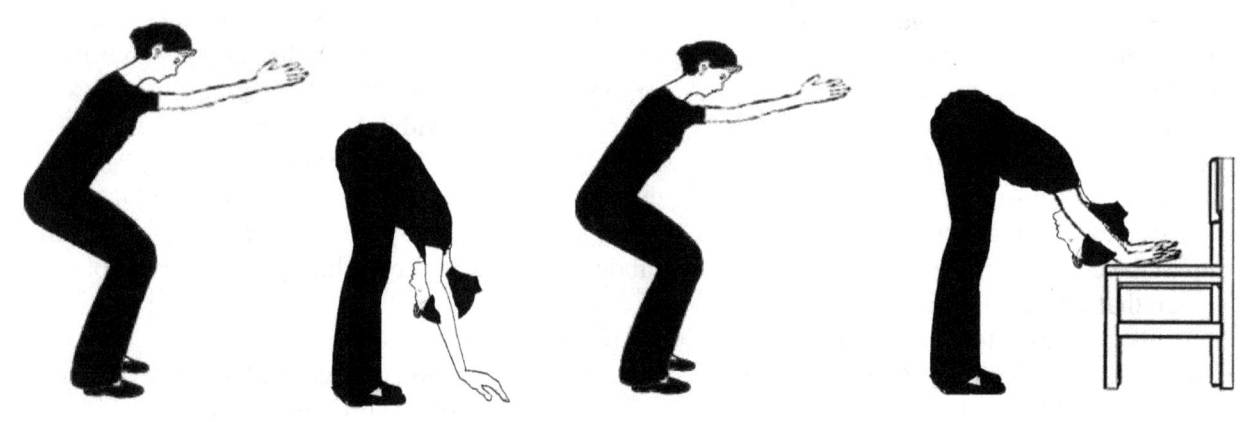

## Lunge

Next step the right foot back so you are in a lunge position. Press the shoulders away from the ears and keep the back straight. Keep the front knee aligned over the ankle.

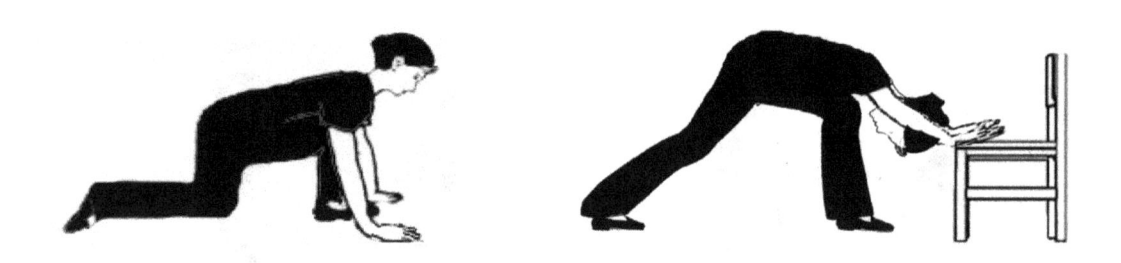

**Downdog**

Step the left foot back, press into your hands, reach the hips back, and lengthen the spine. Do not round the back or lift the shoulders to the ears. Press both heels towards the floor. Keep some weight in the hands in order to provide weight bearing exercise for the wrists and arms.

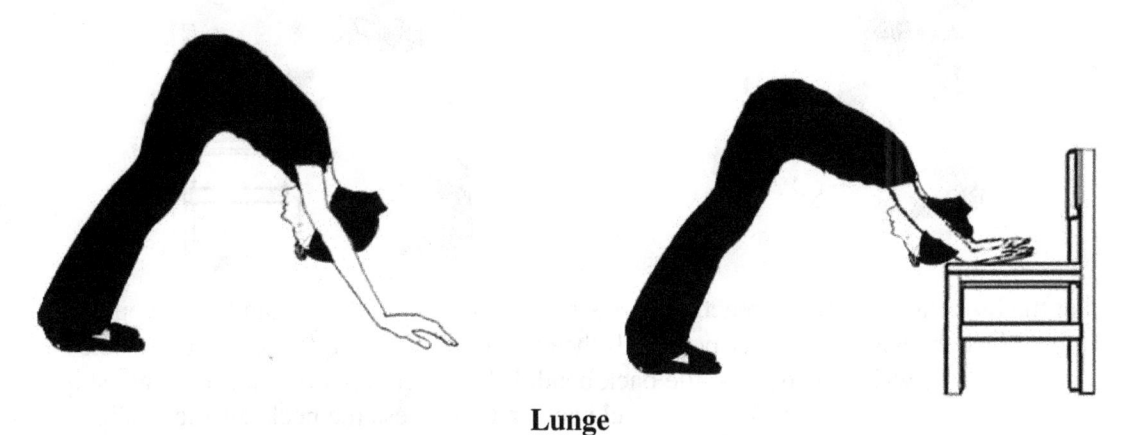

**Lunge**

Next step the right foot forward back into lunge position. Keep the front knee aligned over the ankle.

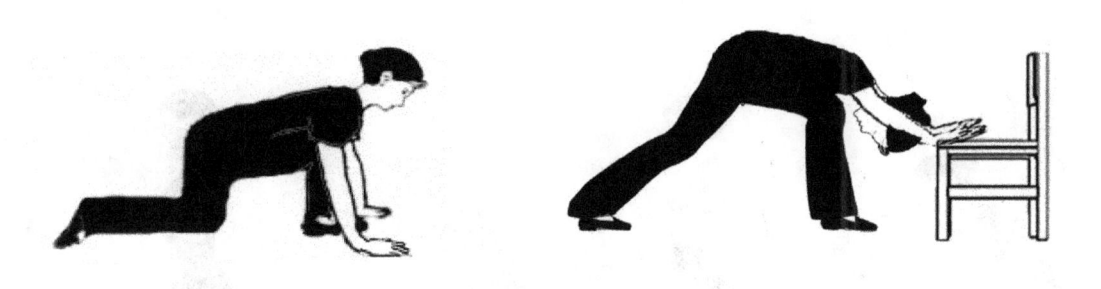

## Forward Bend

Step the feet together and come back to forward bend . Bend your knees as much as you can. This will help to protect the back.

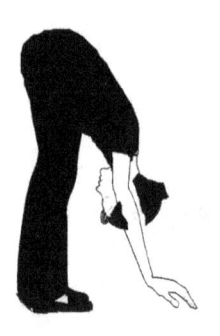

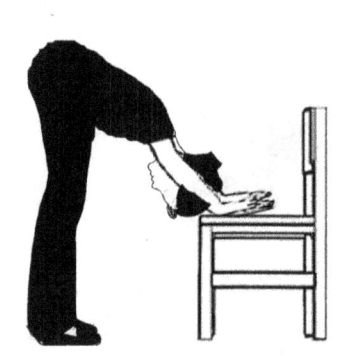

Bend at the hips (hip hinge) and reach the arms forward and come up to standing. Keep the back straight and place the hands in prayer pose. Lift the arms overhead and if it feels appropriate lengthen up from the waist and do a gentle back bend. If back bending does not feel right skip this movement. Make sure you do not drop the head back and compress the neck. Just look slightly up at an angle. Then come back up straight. Lower the arms back to prayer position in front of the heart. Repeat the same sequence on the other leg. Doing both sides is one round of Salutation to the Sun. Repeat as many rounds as feels comfortable.

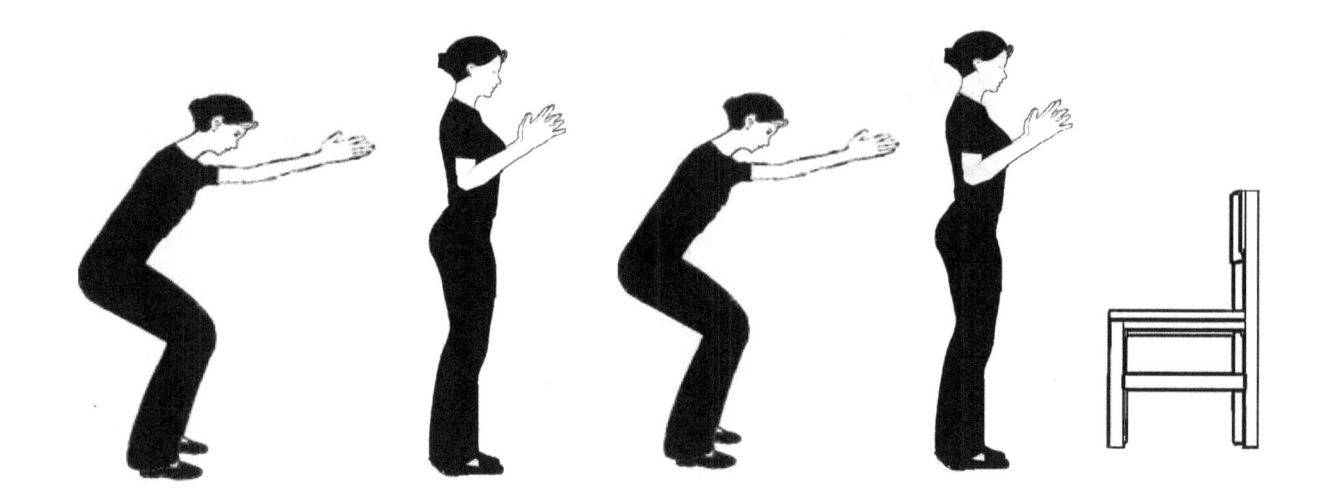

## Warrior III Pose

Check your posture before you begin. Shoulders should be back and down and over the hips. Knees should remain slightly bent. Tuck in the chin and think about pushing the crown of the head up to the ceiling without lifting your chin. The abdominal muscles are lightly pulled in, but not so much that it restricts your breathing.

Without raising the shoulders up, bring your arms up in front of you about shoulder height with the palms facing each other. Begin to lift the right leg up straight behind you. The shoulders can tip *slightly* forward, but keep the body in a straight line from the heel to the head. Keep the natural curve in the low back. Lift the back leg as much as your balance allows. Check that you do not lift the leg so high that you cause discomfort in the low back. The purpose of this posture is to challenge your ability to stand on one foot and should not cause back pain. The left knee (the leg you are standing on) should not be locked. Hold for 5-10 deep belly breaths, or to comfort. Repeat on the left.

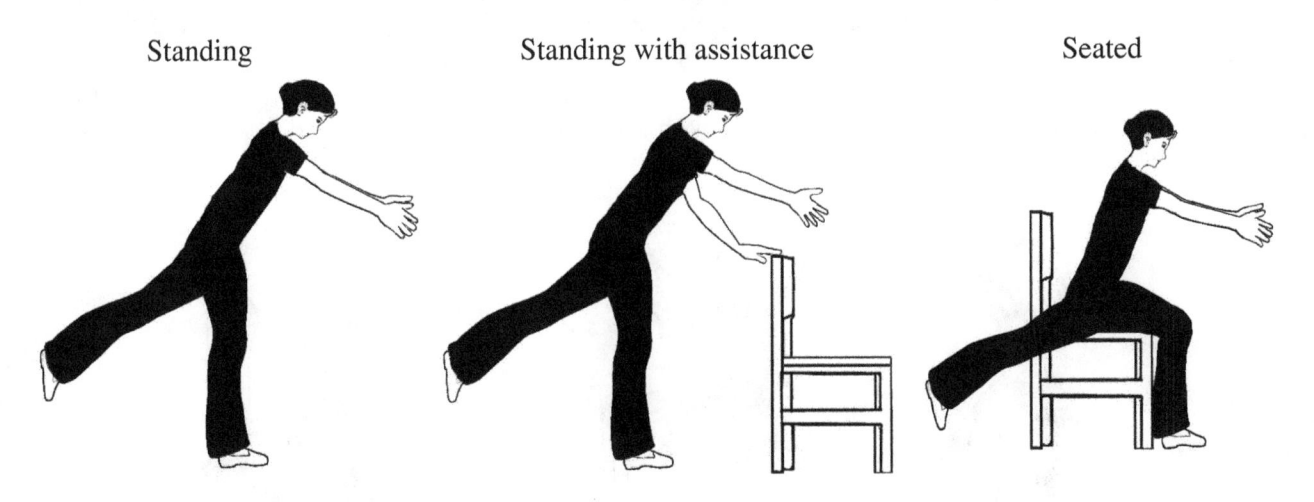

Standing     Standing with assistance     Seated

### Checklist
- Stand or sit up straight
- Keep the shoulders down away from the ears
- Keep the knees slightly bent and the natural curve in the low back
- Do not lift the leg so high that you cause back pain
- Do not drop the shoulders too far forward
- Hold for 5-10 deep belly breaths, or to comfort
- Use diaphragmatic breathing through the nose as much as possible
- Do not exercise to the point of strain or discomfort
- Remember the goal of yoga is to find that point where you are challenging yourself but not struggling

# Tree Pose

Check your posture before you begin. Shoulders should be back and down and over the hips. Knees should remain slightly bent. Tuck in the chin and think about pushing the crown of the head up to the ceiling without lifting your chin. The abdominal muscles are lightly pulled in, but not so much that it restricts your breathing.

Without raising the shoulders up, lift your arms up overhead with the palms facing each other. Shift your weight into the left leg. Begin to bend the right knee and lift the right foot, placing the sole of the right foot against the inside of the left leg. The higher you lift the right foot, the more challenging this posture is. Do not place the right foot directly on the side of the left knee in order to protect the joint. You may wish to start by bringing the right foot to the left ankle bone and keep the right toes on the floor. Bring the hips under the shoulders. Keep the natural curve in the low back. Lift the leg as high as your balance allows. The left knee (the leg you are standing on) should not be locked. Your right foot should be below or above the knee joint. Hold for 5-10 deep belly breaths, or to comfort. Repeat on the left.

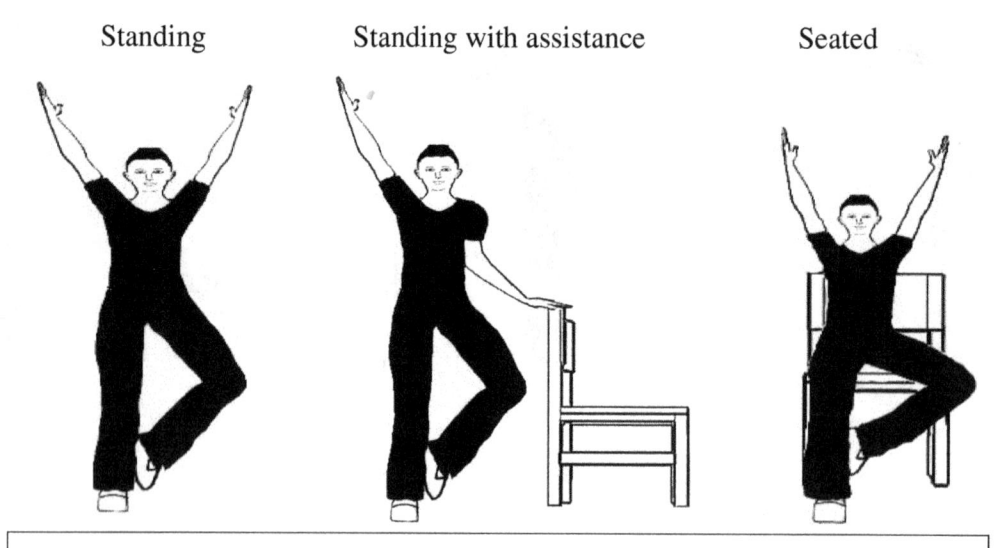

Standing     Standing with assistance     Seated

### Checklist
- ✓ Stand or sit up straight
- ✓ Keep the shoulders down away from the ears
- ✓ Keep the hips under the shoulders
- ✓ Keep the knees slightly bent and the natural curve in the low back
- ✓ Hold for 5-10 deep belly breaths, or to comfort
- ✓ Use diaphragmatic breathing through the nose as much as possible
- ✓ Do not exercise to the point of strain or discomfort
- ✓ Remember the goal of yoga is to find that point where you are challenging yourself but not struggling

## Dancer's Pose/Quadriceps Stretch

Check your posture before you begin. Shoulders should be back and down and over the hips. Knees should remain slightly bent. Tuck in the chin and think about pushing the crown of the head up to the ceiling without lifting your chin. The abdominal muscles are lightly pulled in, but not so much that it restricts your breathing.

Shift your weight into the left leg. Bend the right knee, bringing the heel as close to the buttocks as you can. Bring the hips under the shoulders. Bring the knees together and let the right knee point down towards the floor as much as possible. If it is comfortable to do so, hold onto your right ankle or your right sock or pant leg. If this is creates too deep of a stretch just lift the heel back. Hold for 5-10 deep belly breaths, or to comfort. Repeat on the left.

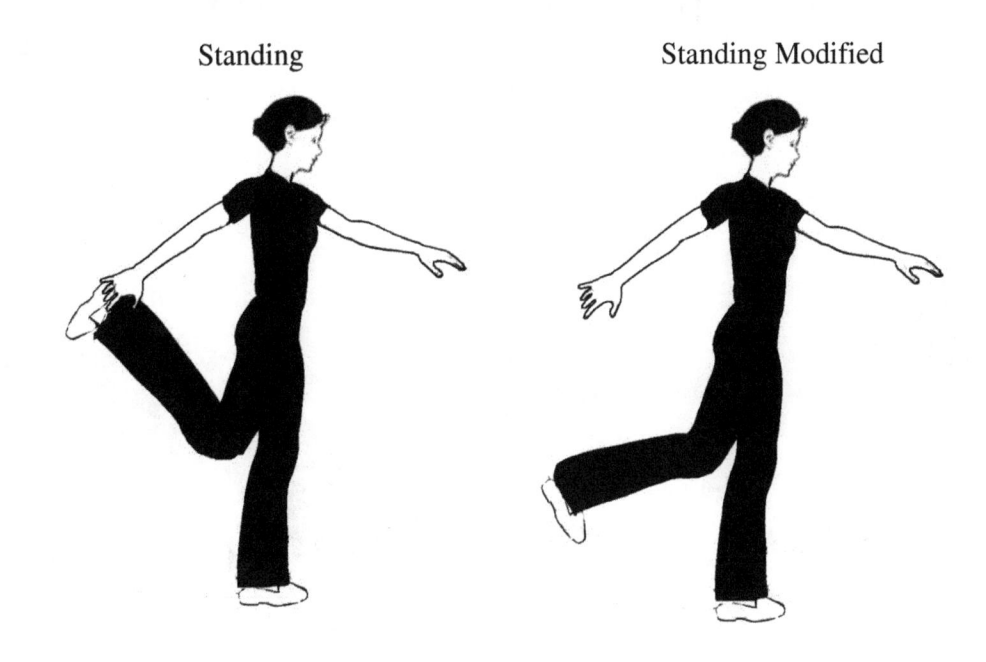

Standing

Standing Modified

Standing with assistance                Seated

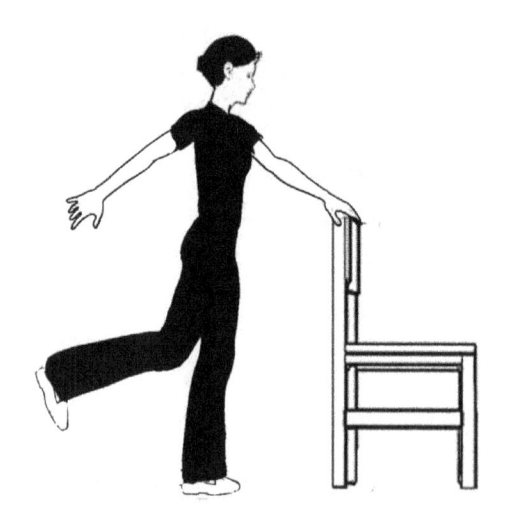

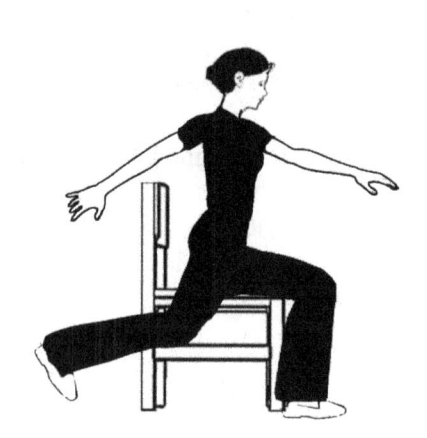

### Checklist
- Stand or sit up straight
- Keep the shoulders down away from the ears
- Keep the hips under the shoulders
- Keep the knees slightly bent and the natural curve in the low back
- Hold for 5-10 deep belly breaths, or to comfort
- Use diaphragmatic breathing through the nose as much as possible
- Do not exercise to the point of strain or discomfort
- Remember the goal of yoga is to find that point where you are challenging yourself but not struggling

## Victory Squat Pose/W Stretch

Check your posture before you begin. Shoulders should be back and down and over the hips. Knees should remain slightly bent. Tuck in the chin and think about pushing the crown of the head up to the ceiling without lifting your chin. The abdominal muscles are lightly pulled in, but not so much that it restricts your breathing.

Without raising the shoulders up, bring the arms into a "W" shape. Bring the hands back so they are in a straight line with the elbows. The legs are in a slight squat position. Keep the natural curve in the low back. Keeping the hands and elbows in line, draw the elbows and hands back as far as you can, squeezing the shoulder blades together in the back. Do not let the head come forward.

This exercise is helpful to correct a forward head and posture. Another variation is to do this stretch with your back against a wall. Stand with the knees slightly bent, with the buttocks and back against the wall. If possible let the back of the head touch the wall, keeping the chin parallel to the floor. Do not tilt your head back to make it touch. If your head does not touch, just come back as far as you can. With consistent stretching you may eventually be able to go back further. Keeping the hands and elbows in line, draw the elbows and hands back as close to the wall as you can. Hold for 5-10 deep belly breaths, or to comfort. Repeat on the left.

Standing front view

Standing back view.
Bring the shoulder blades together

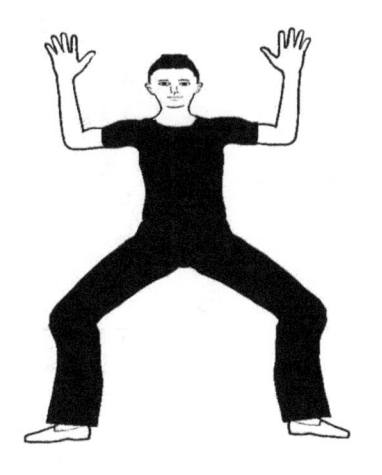

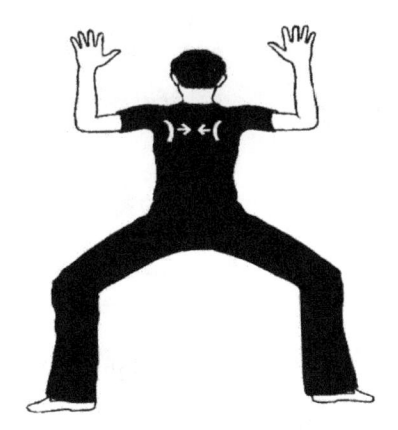

Against a wall          Seated

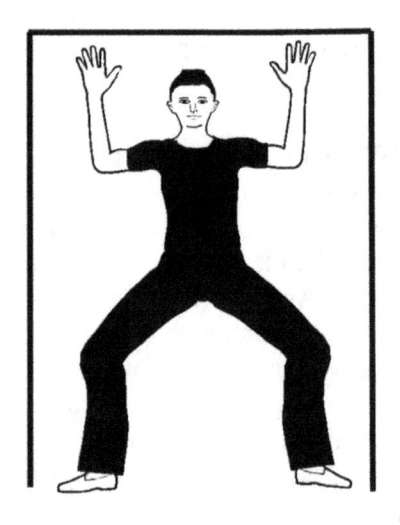

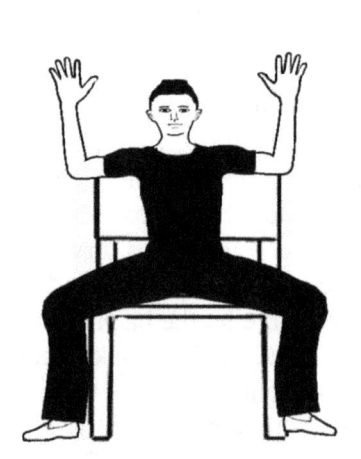

### Checklist
- Stand or sit up straight
- Keep the shoulders down away from the ears
- Keep the hips under the shoulders
- Keep the knees slightly bent and the natural curve in the low back
- Hold for 5-10 deep belly breaths, or to comfort
- Use diaphragmatic breathing through the nose as much as possible
- Do not exercise to the point of strain or discomfort
- Remember the goal of yoga is to find that point where you are challenging yourself but not struggling

## Chest Stretch

This movement will help to open the chest and the shoulders and it is helpful for correcting posture. This stretch is good after working at a desk or computer for some time.

Check your posture before you begin. Shoulders should be back and down and over the hips. Knees should remain slightly bent. Tuck the chin in and think about pushing the crown of the head up to the ceiling without lifting your chin. The abdominal muscles are lightly pulled in, but not so much as to restrict your breathing.

If you can, clasp your hands behind your back. If you are unable to clasp your hands, just reach back. Keep your knees slightly bent. Draw your shoulder blades together and lift your hands away from your body as far as you can without hurting your shoulders. Be careful to not lean forward as you lift your hands. Your shoulders should stay over your hips. Move gently and slowly, counting *one-one thousand, two-one thousand, three-one thousand, four-one thousand* to lift your arms, and use the same count to lower the arms down. Repeat 8-12 times.

Standing　　　　　　　　　　　Seated

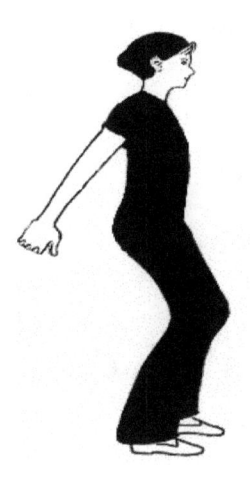

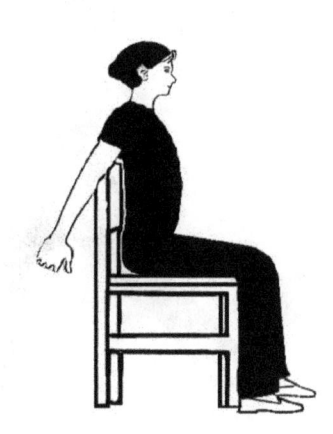

### Checklist
- ✓ Stand up straight
- ✓ Move slowly using a "4 thousand count" for each movement
- ✓ Use diaphragmatic breathing through the nose as much as possible
- ✓ Keep the knees slightly bent when standing
- ✓ Keep the natural arch in the low back
- ✓ Do not lean forward as you lift the arms
- ✓ Do not exercise to the point of strain or discomfort

## Hamstring Stretch/Seated Forward Bend Pose

Check your posture before you begin. Shoulders should be back and down and over the hips. Knees should remain slightly bent. Tuck in the chin and think about pushing the crown of the head up to the ceiling without lifting your chin. The abdominal muscles are lightly pulled in, but not so much that it restricts your breathing.

Step your right foot forward into a lunge position. The back knee is straight but not locked, and the front knee is bent. Both feet and toes are facing forward. Make sure that your right knee does not extend past your right ankle bone. You should be able to look down at your right knee and see both your right toes and the arch of the right foot. If you need a deeper stretch step the feet wider apart rather then bringing the right knee beyond the toes. This will help to protect the knee joint from injury. Bring the hips under the shoulders. Press your back heel down to the floor, but be careful to not lock the back knee. Hold for 5-10 deep belly breaths, or to comfort. Repeat with the right leg back.

Standing

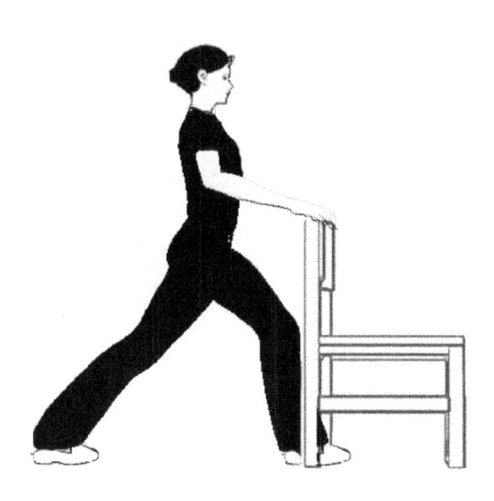

## Seated

Sit at the front edge of the chair. Extend your right leg forward and pull the toes towards you. Keep the back straight and bring your chest forward, hinging at the hips. Do not round your back or slump forward.

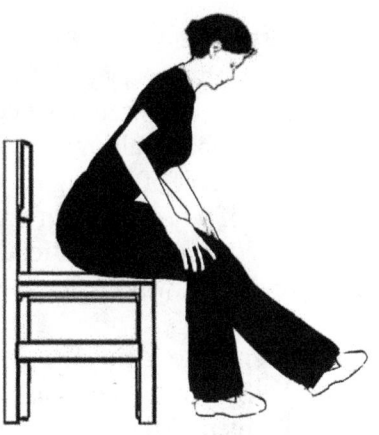

### Checklist
- ✓ Stand or sit up straight
- ✓ Keep the shoulders down away from the ears
- ✓ Keep the hips under the shoulders
- ✓ Keep the knees slightly bent and the natural curve in the low back
- ✓ Hold for 5-10 deep belly breaths, or to comfort
- ✓ Use diaphragmatic breathing through the nose as much as possible
- ✓ Do not exercise to the point of strain or discomfort
- ✓ Remember the goal of yoga is to find that point where you are challenging yourself but not struggling

## Seated and Floor Postures

The next series of poses can either be done seated or on the floor. Listen to your body to determine which option is best for you.

## Floor Exercises

On days when you feel able floor exercises can be very beneficial for those with osteoporosis. The floor is a solid surface that provides feedback as to whether or not the back is straight and allows you to stretch deeply as you do not have to worry about falling.

Doing floor exercises also keeps you in the habit of getting up and down. You may find that you will be able to get up more easily after a fall if you have been practicing getting up from the floor. Performing these exercises on a couch or bed is not as beneficial as these surfaces are often too soft and do not provide enough support, however as always listen to your body and do what is best for you.

When performing floor exercises it is essential to maintain a pelvic tilt in order to protect the back from injury. Letting your back arch off the floor can lead to back strain. It is also very important to keep your neck straight and in correct alignment. To prevent neck strain place a towel or pillow under the head so the neck remains straight. However, do not use too high of a pillow as that will push the head forward. It is best to have someone help you get set up the first time so they can see if your neck is straight and to help you decide how much cushioning you need under your head.

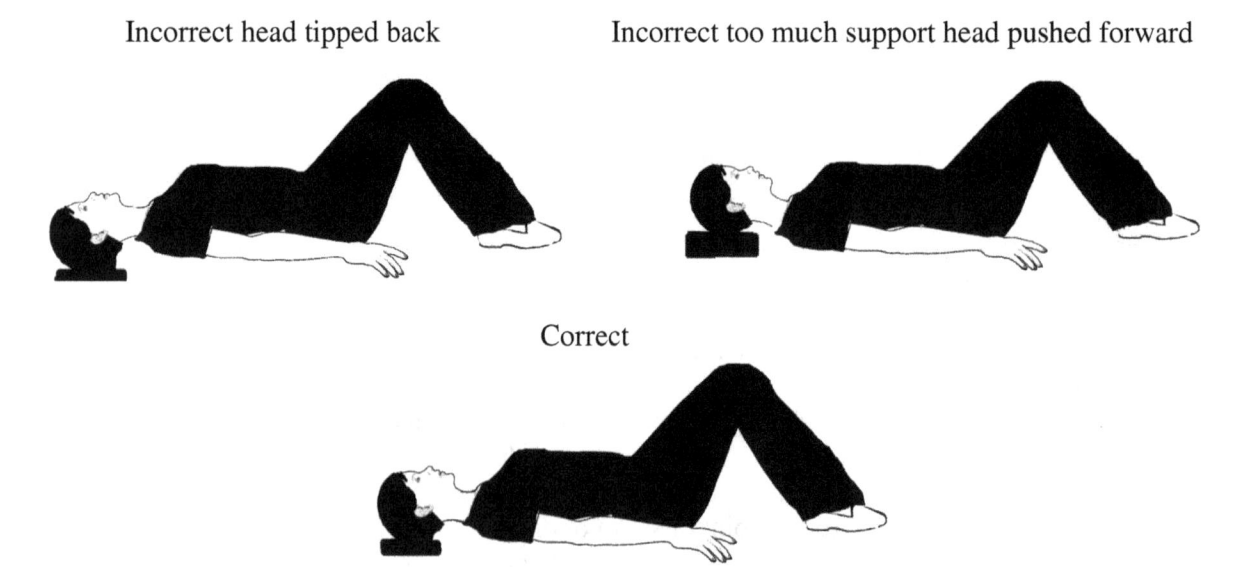

Incorrect head tipped back      Incorrect too much support head pushed forward

Correct

## Pelvic Tilts

Lie on the floor on your back with the knees bent, feet on the floor. Make sure you keep the head and neck level, do not arch the head or tip the chin back. If you find that you are arching your neck, place a pillow under the head.

This exercise helps to strengthen the abdominal muscles. Without lifting the hips or buttocks, press your low back down into the floor. Try to slip your hands under your low back. If you are doing this exercise correctly you should feel your low back tight against the floor, and you should not be able to get your hands under your back. Hold for a slow count of five. Then relax and let the low back arch enough so that you can slip your hands under your back. Repeat 8-12 times.

Pressing the low back flat.     Letting the low back arch.

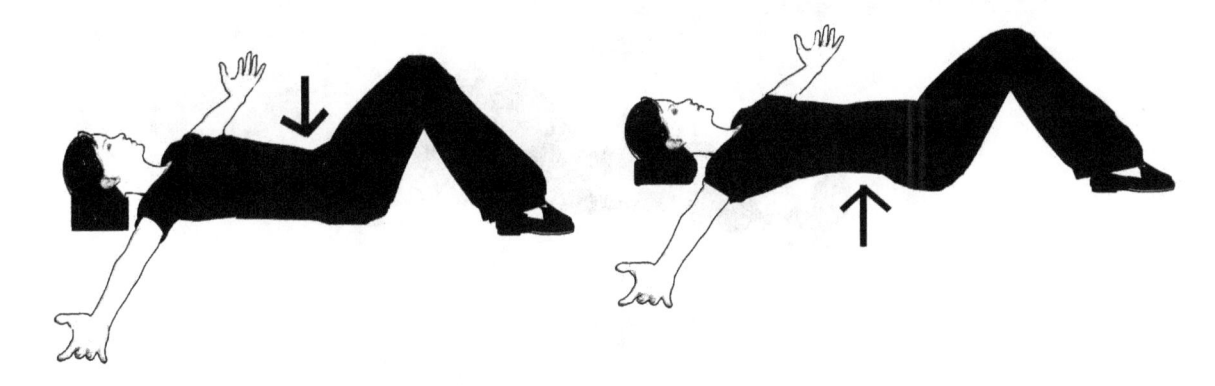

### Checklist
- ✓ Make sure you keep your head and chin level
- ✓ Make sure you are moving the just the low back and not lifting the hips or buttocks
- ✓ Use diaphragmatic breathing through the nose as much as possible
- ✓ Do not exercise to the point of strain or discomfort
- ✓ Remember the goal of yoga is to find that point where you are challenging yourself but not struggling

# Bridge

This posture is only shown on the floor as there are no comparable seated versions. If you are unable to do floor exercises skip ahead to the next page. Lie on the floor on your back with the knees bent, feet on the floor. Make sure you keep the head and neck level do not arch the head or tip the chin back. If you find that you are arching your neck, place a pillow under the head.

Tighten the buttocks muscles and lift the hips off the floor as high as you can. Make sure you do not let the head tip back as you lift, keep the neck straight and the chin level. Keep both knees pointing straight up to the ceiling do not let the knees roll in or out. Exhale as you lift the hips and inhale as you lower the hips. Repeat 8-12 times.

After completing 8-12 repetitions hold for a stretch in the lifted position for 5-10 deep belly breaths, or to comfort.

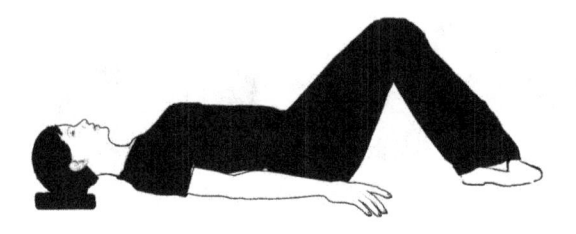

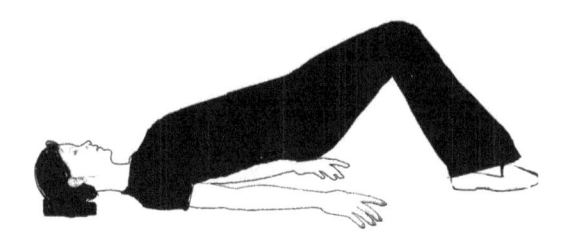

### Checklist
- ✓ Make sure you keep your head and chin level
- ✓ Make sure you do not tip the head back when you lift the hips
- ✓ Keep the knees pointing up to the ceiling
- ✓ Use diaphragmatic breathing through the nose as much as possible
- ✓ Do not exercise to the point of strain or discomfort
- ✓ Remember the goal of yoga is to find that point where you are challenging yourself but not struggling

## Knee To Chest Pose

If you have moderate to severe osteoporosis, a history of compression fractures, or if you have experienced a postural change or loss of height, check with your healthcare provider about the appropriateness of this movement. Check your posture before you begin. Shoulders should be back and down and over the hips. Tuck in the chin and think about pushing the crown of the head up to the ceiling without lifting your chin. The abdominal muscles are lightly pulled in, but not so much that it restricts your breathing.

### Seated

Sit towards the front edge of the chair and lean your upper back against the chair. Draw your right knee up towards your chest and if possible hold underneath the knee. Be careful not to hold in front of the knee as this can compress the joint. If you can not reach your right knee, wrap a towel or strap under the foot and hold the ends with your hands. *Do not pull the leg in hard, just bring the knee in enough until you feel a gentle stretch.* Hold for 5-10 deep belly breaths, or to comfort. Repeat with the left knee.

Holding under knee.

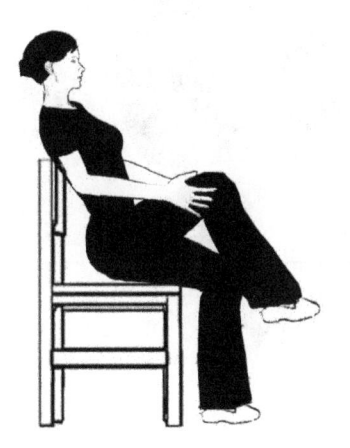

Modification with towel.

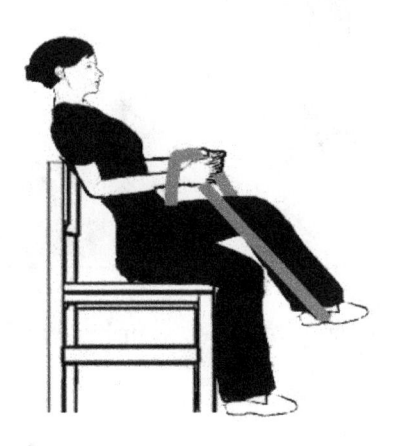

## Floor variation

Lie on the floor on your back. Keep the head and neck level. If you find that you are arching your neck, place a pillow under the head. Begin with a pelvic tilt. Throughout this exercise make sure your low back stays in contact with the floor.

Without arching the back bring your right knee towards your chest. You can either hold the knee with your hands or wrap a towel or yoga strap around the knee. When holding the knee make sure you hold under the knee and not on top of the knee so you do not compress the joint. Make sure your head stays on the floor or pillow.

Do not hold the head off the floor just to reach your knee as this strains the neck. *Do not pull the leg in hard, just bring the knee in enough until you feel a gentle stretch in the back of the leg you are holding up.* Hold for five to ten deep belly breaths or for as long as is comfortable. Repeat with the other leg.

Knee To Chest           Knee To Chest With Towel

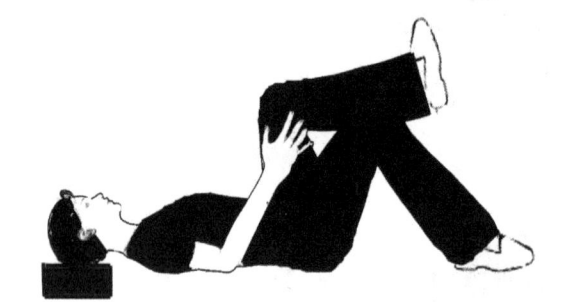

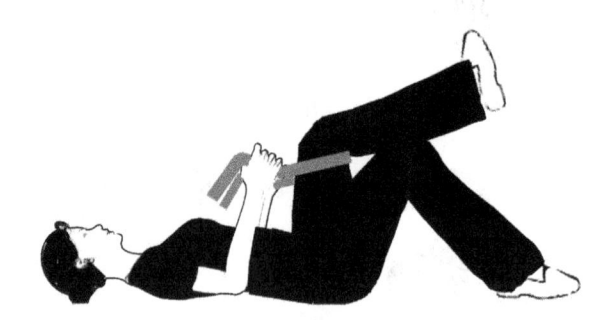

### Checklist
- ✓ Make sure you keep your head and chin level and your head on the floor or pillow
- ✓ Make sure you keep the low back in contact with the floor
- ✓ Keep the shoulders down away from the ears
- ✓ Make sure you hold on underneath the knee, not in front of the knee
- ✓ Hold for 5-10 deep belly breaths, or to comfort
- ✓ Use diaphragmatic breathing through the nose as much as possible
- ✓ Do not exercise to the point of strain or discomfort
- ✓ Remember the goal of yoga is to find that point where you are challenging yourself but not struggling

## Seated Spinal Twist Pose

Check your posture before you begin. Shoulders should be back and down and over the hips. Tuck in the chin and think about pushing the crown of the head up to the ceiling without lifting your chin. The abdominal muscles are lightly pulled in, but not so much that it restricts your breathing.

Use caution with this posture if you have severe osteoporosis or compression fractures. Twisting motions may be contraindicated. Check with your health care provider if you have concerns about the appropriateness of twisting movements.

Sit up straight away from the back of the chair if possible. Reach the left hand to the outside of the right knee. Turn to the right beginning the movement at the waist. Reach your right arm back behind you and look over your right shoulder. Turn as far as you comfortably can and look behind you as far as you can. You can press *gently* against your knee to help you twist further. Each time you inhale sit up straighter. Each time you exhale turn from the waist a little bit more. Hold for five to ten deep belly breaths, or for as long as is comfortable. Repeat with the right hand on the outside of the left knee.

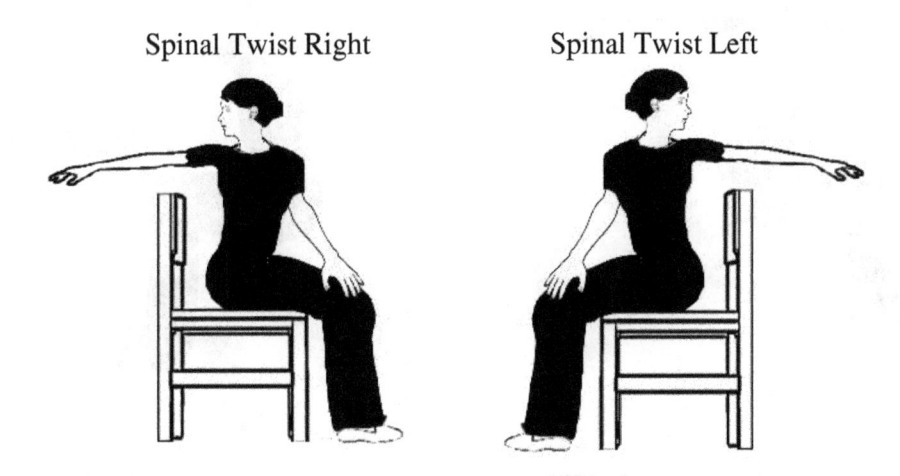

Spinal Twist Right        Spinal Twist Left

### Checklist
- ✓ Sit up straight and away from the back of the chair as much as possible
- ✓ Keep the shoulders down away from the ears
- ✓ Keep the natural curve in the low back
- ✓ Use caution if you have back sensitivities
- ✓ Hold for five to ten deep belly breaths, or to comfort
- ✓ Use diaphragmatic breathing through the nose as much as possible
- ✓ Do not exercise to the point of strain or discomfort
- ✓ Remember the goal of yoga is to find that point where you are challenging yourself but not struggling

## Floor variation

Be gentle with this movement if you have any back injuries. Lie on the floor on your back with the knees bent, feet on the floor. Make sure you keep the head and neck level do not arch the head or tip the chin back. If you find that you are arching your neck, place a pillow under the head.

Bring your arms out to the side in a "T" position with the palms facing the ceiling. Slowly lower both knees to one side and let the knees come as close to the floor as possible. If that bothers your back stay in a pelvic tilt and do not drop the knees as far down. Looking away from the knees is a deeper stretch, looking towards the knees is a gentler stretch. Otherwise look straight up or towards your knees. Hold for five to ten deep belly breaths or for as long as is comfortable. Repeat other side.

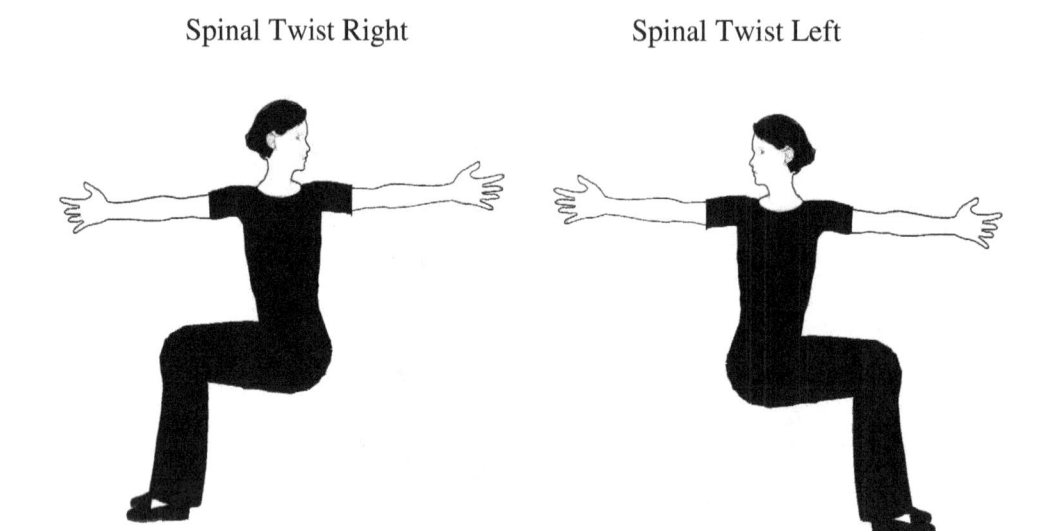

Spinal Twist Right    Spinal Twist Left

### Checklist
- ✓ Make sure you keep your head and chin level and your head on the floor or pillow
- ✓ Only twist as far as it is comfortable to do so – use caution if your back is sensitive
- ✓ Use diaphragmatic breathing through the nose as much as possible
- ✓ Do not exercise to the point of strain or discomfort
- ✓ Remember the goal of yoga is to find that point where you are challenging yourself but not struggling

## Single Arm Overhead Reach

If lying on the floor is uncomfortable these next few exercises can be done against a wall.

### Standing

Stand one to two feet away from the wall. Lean back so that the buttocks, both shoulder blades and the back of the head are all touching the wall. Do not tip the head back just to touch the head. Keep the chin level and just draw he chin back as far as you are able. With regular stretching you may find that eventually your head will touch.

Bring your right arm overhead with the palm facing out. Bring your arm as close as you can to the wall without over arching the low back. Keep the elbow close to the ear when the arm is up. Then bring the arm back down repeat with the left arm. Do eight to twelve repetitions. One repetition involves going to both sides.

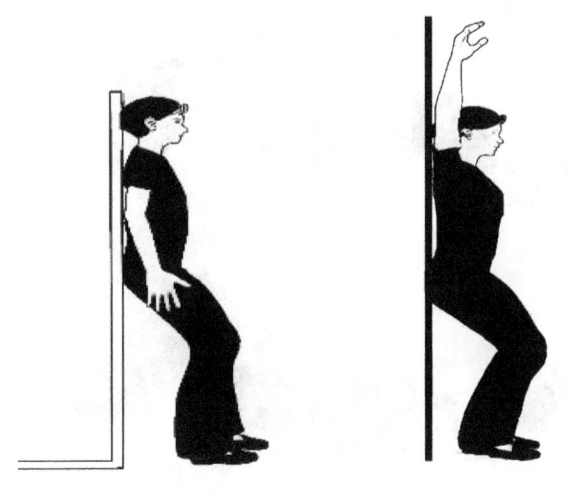

Checklist
- ✓ Make sure you keep your head and chin level
- ✓ Avoid over arching the low back
- ✓ Use diaphragmatic breathing through the nose as much as possible
- ✓ Do not exercise to the point of strain or discomfort
- ✓ Remember the goal of yoga is to find that point where you are challenging yourself but not struggling

## Floor Variation

Lie on the floor on your back with the knees bent, feet on the floor. Make sure you keep the head and neck level using a pillow if necessary. Begin with a pelvic tilt. Throughout this exercise make sure your low back stays in contact with the floor. Do not let the low back arch. If you are dealing with shoulder injuries use caution with the next two postures.

Keeping the low back tight against the floor bring your right arm overhead with the palm facing up. Bring your arm as close as you can to the floor keeping your low back pressed into the floor. Keep the elbow close to the ear when the arm is back. If the back begins to arch make the movement smaller. The further away from the floor that your arm is the easier it is to keep your back flat. You will find that as your abdominal muscles strengthen and your shoulders become more flexible you will be able to lower your arm closer to the floor. Then bring the arm back and repeat with the left arm. Do eight to twelve repetitions. One repetition involves going to both sides.

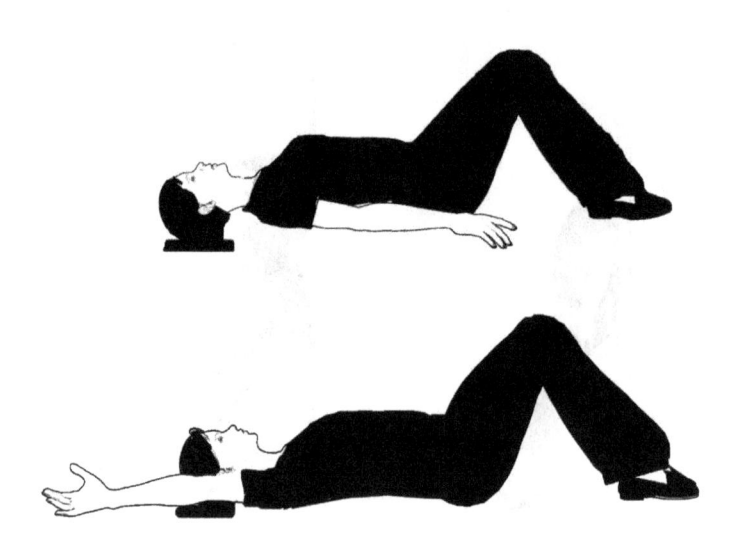

---

### Checklist
- ✓ Make sure you keep your head and chin level
- ✓ Make sure you keep the low back in contact with the floor
- ✓ Use diaphragmatic breathing through the nose as much as possible
- ✓ Do not exercise to the point of strain or discomfort
- ✓ Remember the goal of yoga is to find that point where you are challenging yourself but not struggling

## Double Arm Overhead Reach
Standing

Stand one to two feet away from the wall. Lean back so that the buttocks, both shoulder blades and the back of the head are all touching the wall. Do not tip the head back just to touch the head. Keep the chin level and just draw he chin back as far as you are able. With regular stretching you may find that eventually your head will touch.

Clasp your hands and lift them both up overhead and bring the hands as close as you can to the wall without over arching the low back. Keep the elbows close to the ears when the arms are up. Then bring the arm back down repeat with the left arm. Do eight to twelve repetitions.

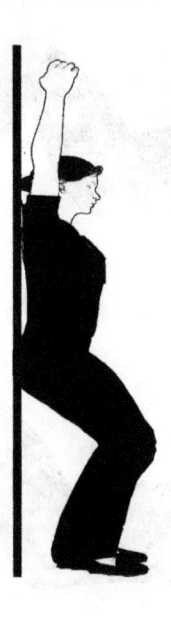

Checklist
- ✓ Make sure you keep your head and chin level
- ✓ Avoid over arching the low back
- ✓ Use diaphragmatic breathing through the nose as much as possible
- ✓ Do not exercise to the point of strain or discomfort
- ✓ Remember the goal of yoga is to find that point where you are challenging yourself but not struggling

## Floor Variation

Clasp the hands and reach both arms up straight. Slowly bring your arms as close as you can to the floor keeping your low back pressed into the floor. Keep the elbows close to the ears when the arms are back. Then slowly lift the arms back up. If the back begins to arch make the movement smaller. Do eight to twelve repetitions. After completing eight to twelve repetitions hold for a stretch with both arms back and the back flat on the floor. Hold for five to ten deep belly breaths, or to comfort.

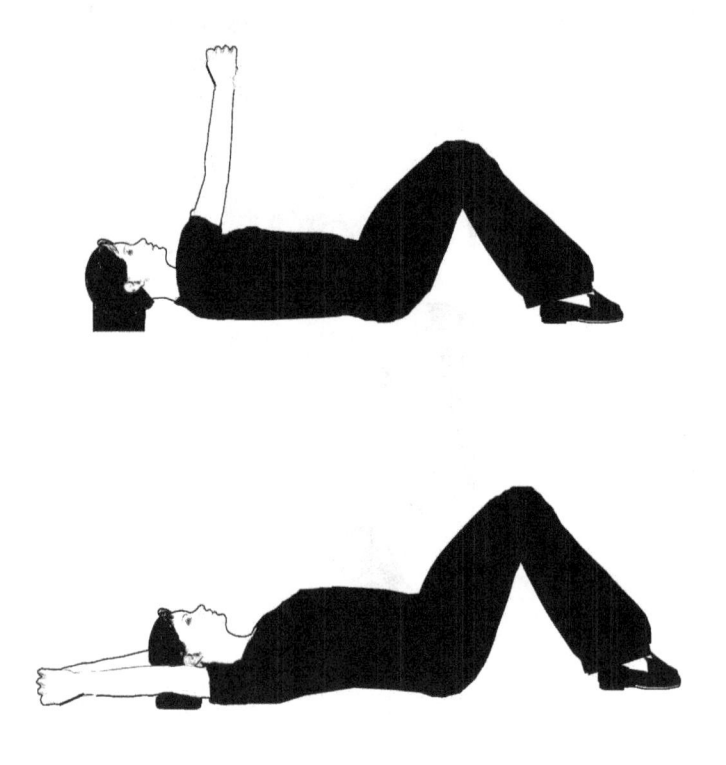

### Checklist
- ✓ Make sure you keep your head and chin level
- ✓ Keep the low back pressed into the floor
- ✓ Use diaphragmatic breathing through the nose as much as possible
- ✓ Do not exercise to the point of strain or discomfort
- ✓ Remember the goal of yoga is to find that point where you are challenging yourself but not struggling

## Opposite Arm To Leg Reach

### Standing

Stand one to two feet away from the wall. Lean back so that the buttocks, both shoulder blades and the back of the head are all touching the wall. Do not tip the head back just to touch the head. Keep the chin level and just draw the chin back as far as you are able. With regular stretching you may find that eventually your head will touch.

Lift the right hand up and bring the back of the hand as close as you can to the wall. Tighten the stomach muscles and bring the right hand down to shoulder height as you lift the left leg straight up to the front. Keep the back of the head, shoulder blades and buttocks against the wall. Then bring the arm back up and lower the leg down. Repeat with the left arm and right leg. Do eight to twelve repetitions. One repetition is both sides.

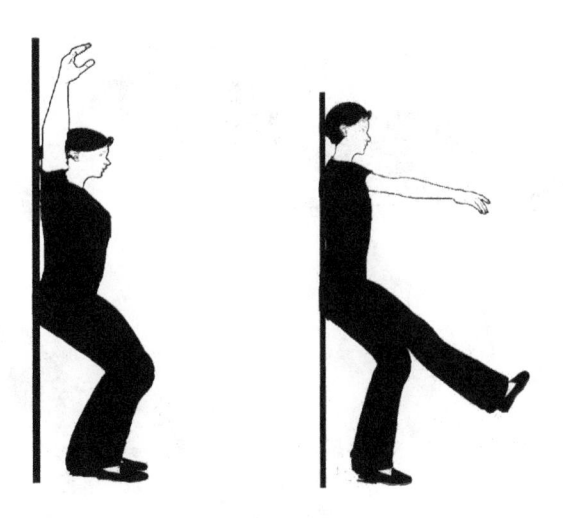

Checklist
- ✓ Make sure you keep your head and chin level
- ✓ Avoid over arching the low back
- ✓ Use diaphragmatic breathing through the nose as much as possible
- ✓ Do not exercise to the point of strain or discomfort
- ✓ Remember the goal of yoga is to find that point where you are challenging yourself but not struggling

## Floor variation

Lie on the floor on your back with the knees bent, feet on the floor. Keep the head and neck level using a pillow if necessary. Begin with a pelvic tilt. Throughout this exercise make sure your low back stays in contact with the floor. Do not let the low back arch.

Keeping the low back tight against the floor bring your right arm overhead and stretch your left leg out straight. Keep your right knee bent and the right foot on the floor. Bring your arm and leg as close as you can to the floor keeping your low back pressed into the floor. If the back begins to arch make the movement smaller. The further away from the floor that your arm and leg is, the easier it is to keep your back flat. You will find that as your abdominal muscles strengthen you will be able to lower your arm and leg closer to the floor.

Then bring the arm and leg all the way back. Repeat with the left arm and right leg. Keep the left knee bent and the left foot on the floor. Do eight to twelve repetitions. One repetition involves going to both sides.

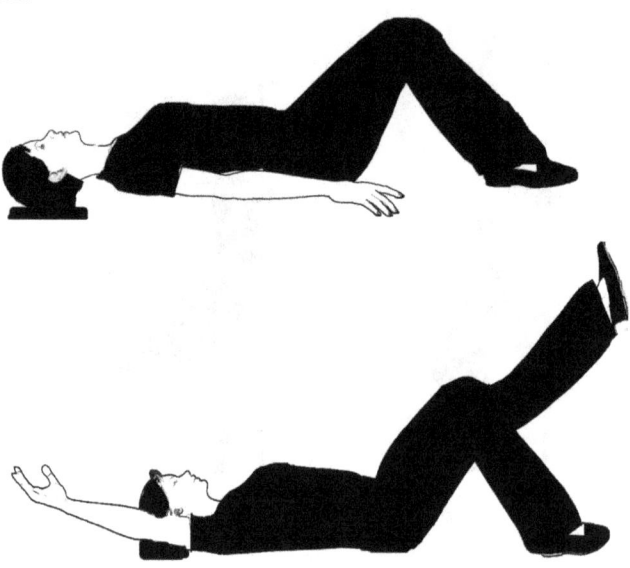

| Checklist |
| --- |
| ✓ Make sure you keep your head and chin level |
| ✓ Keep the low back pressed into the floor |
| ✓ Use diaphragmatic breathing through the nose as much as possible |
| ✓ Do not exercise to the point of strain or discomfort |
| ✓ Remember the goal of yoga is to find that point where you are challenging yourself but not struggling |

The next series of exercises are shown lying on the stomach. However, they can also be done standing and facing a wall. Many of us spend much of our day with the shoulders rounded forward as we go about daily tasks. This can cause the upper back muscles to become weak and over-stretched and the chest muscles to become tight. These postures are beneficial to help strengthen the upper back muscles and stretch the chest muscles to help correct posture.

Be gentle if your back is sensitive. You can modify these postures by placing a pillow under the hips which will lessen the arch in the low back. You may find that at first you need to use a pillow and then as the back strengthens you can do the postures without the pillow. Another modification is to place a rolled towel under the forehead if you find that lying with the face down is uncomfortable.

### Single Arm Lift

Stand about one to two feet away from the wall, facing the wall. Tighten the abdominal and buttocks muscles to protect the back. Place both hands against the wall overhead and about hip width apart. Then lift the right arm off the wall and back as far as you can without hurting your shoulders or arching your back. Then lower the right hand back to the wall and repeat with the left hand. Do 8 to 12 repetitions with both arms.

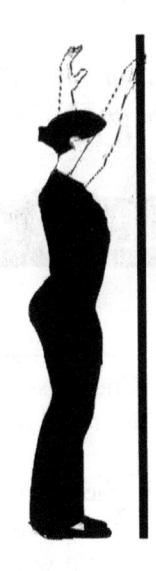

Checklist
- ✓ Only bring the arm back as far as you can without hurting the shoulder
- ✓ Avoid over arching the low back
- ✓ Use diaphragmatic breathing through the nose as much as possible
- ✓ Do not exercise to the point of strain or discomfort
- ✓ Remember the goal of yoga is to find that point where you are challenging yourself but not struggling

## Floor variation

Lie on your stomach with the hands overhead, palms facing the floor, and feet relaxed. Place your forehead or chin on the floor. To protect the neck it is not recommended that you turn your head to the side. If needed you can place a pillow under the hips or a towel roll under the forehead. Press your abdominal muscles and pelvic bones down into the floor and tighten the buttocks muscles. This will help to protect the back.

Lift just the right arm straight up off the floor. The elbow should be near your ear. Do not let the arm drift off to the side. Squeeze the shoulders blades together. Keep your other hand and both feet relaxed on the floor. Keep the head on the floor. One objective of this posture is to learn to work only one area of your body at a time while being able to relax the rest of your body. Try to avoid tightening the muscles of your left arm or lifting the legs off the floor. Hold for 5-10 deep belly breaths or to comfort. Relax and repeat with the left arm.

*Lying flat*  *Lying with a pillow under the hips*

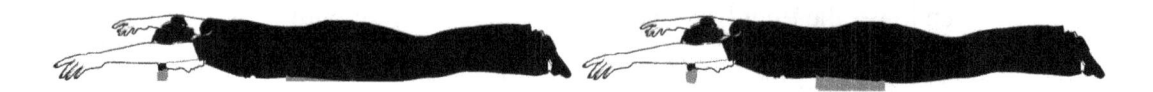

*Lift Just the right arm off the floor.*
*A towel can be placed under the forehead if needed.*

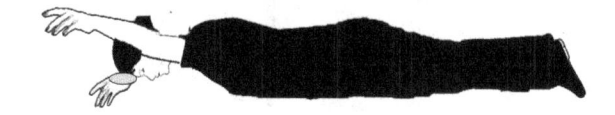

---

### Checklist
- ✓ Press the stomach and hips into the floor and tighten the buttocks muscles to protect the back
- ✓ Lift just one arm at a time. Do not lift the other arm, feet, or head off the floor
- ✓ Use a pillow under the hips &/or towel roll under the forehead if needed
- ✓ Use diaphragmatic breathing through the nose as much as possible
- ✓ Do not exercise to the point of strain or discomfort
- ✓ Remember the goal of yoga is to find that point where you are challenging yourself but not struggling

## Single Leg Lift

Stand about one to two feet away from the wall, facing the wall. Tighten the abdominal and buttocks muscles to protect the back. Place the hands against the wall overhead and about about shoulder width apart. Lift the right leg back as high as possible without hurting the low back. Then lower back down. Do 8 to 12 repetitions then repeat with the left arm.

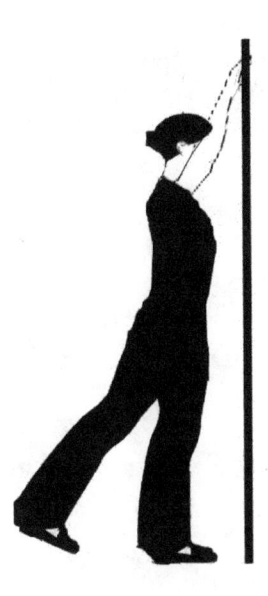

| Checklist |
|---|
| ✓ Only lift the leg as far as you can without hurting the shoulder |
| ✓ Avoid over arching the low back |
| ✓ Use diaphragmatic breathing through the nose as much as possible |
| ✓ Do not exercise to the point of strain or discomfort |
| ✓ Remember the goal of yoga is to find that point where you are challenging yourself but not struggling |

## Floor variation

Lie on your stomach with the hands overhead, palms facing the floor, and feet relaxed. Place your forehead or chin on the floor. To protect the neck it is not recommended that you turn your head to the side. If needed you can place a pillow under the hips or a towel roll under the forehead. Press your abdominal muscles and pelvic bones down into the floor and tighten the buttocks muscles. This will help to protect the back.

Lift just the right leg straight up off the floor. Keep the leg and knee as straight as you can. Keep your other leg and both arms relaxed on the floor. Keep the head on the floor. Squeeze the buttocks muscles as you lift. You should not feel any strain in your low back. Only lift the leg as high as you can without hurting your back. One objective of this posture is to learn to work only one area of your body at a time while being able to relax the rest of your body. Try to avoid tightening the muscles of your left leg or lifting the arms off the floor. Hold for 5-10 deep belly breaths or to comfort. Relax and repeat with the left leg.

*Lying flat*  *Lying with pillow under hips*

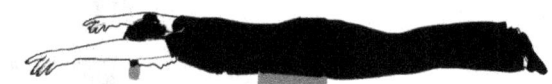

*Lift just the right leg off the floor.*
*A towel can be placed under the forehead if needed.*

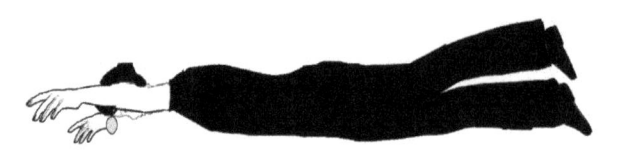

---

### Checklist
- ✓ Press the stomach and hips into the floor and tighten the buttocks muscles to protect the back
- ✓ Lift just one leg at a time. Do not lift the other leg, arms, or head off the floor
- ✓ Use a pillow under the hips &/or towel roll under the forehead if needed
- ✓ Do not lift the leg too high and strain the low back
- ✓ Use diaphragmatic breathing through the nose as much as possible
- ✓ Do not exercise to the point of strain or discomfort
- ✓ Remember the goal of yoga is to find that point where you are challenging yourself but not struggling

## Half Boat Pose

Stand about one to two feet away from the wall, facing the wall. Tighten the abdominal and buttocks muscles to protect the back. Place the hands against the wall overhead and about about shoulder width apart. Lift the right arm off the wall and at the same time lift the left leg back. Then lower the arm and leg back down. Repeat with the left arm and right leg. Do 8 to 12 repetitions. One repetition is going to both sides.

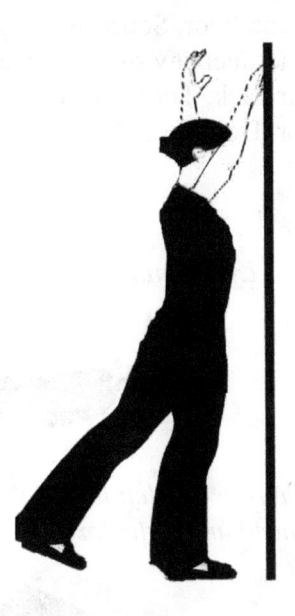

---

Checklist
- ✓ Only lift the arm and leg as far as you can without hurting the shoulder or low back
- ✓ Avoid over arching the low back
- ✓ Use diaphragmatic breathing through the nose as much as possible
- ✓ Do not exercise to the point of strain or discomfort
- ✓ Remember the goal of yoga is to find that point where you are challenging yourself but not struggling

## Floor Variation

Lie on your stomach with the hands overhead, palms facing the floor, and feet relaxed. Place your forehead or chin on the floor. To protect the neck it is not recommended that you turn your head to the side. If needed you can place a pillow under the hips or a towel roll under the forehead. Press your abdominal muscles and pelvic bones down into the floor and tighten the buttocks muscles. This will help to protect the back.

Lift the right arm and left leg straight up off the floor. The right elbow should be near your ear. Do not let the arm drift off to the side. Keep the knee as straight as you can. Keep your left arm and right leg relaxed on the floor. Keep the head on the floor. Squeeze the shoulders blades together and tighten the buttocks muscles. You should not feel any strain in your low back. Only lift the arm and leg as high as you can without hurting your back. Try to avoid tightening the muscles of your left arm or right leg or lifting them off the floor. Hold for 5-10 deep belly breaths or to comfort. Relax and repeat with the left arm and right leg.

*Lying flat*    *Lying with pillow under hips*

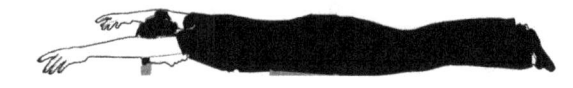

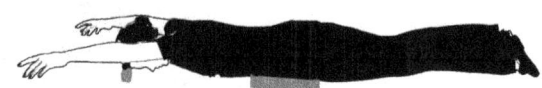

*Lift just the right arm and left leg off the floor.*
*A towel can be placed under the forehead if needed.*

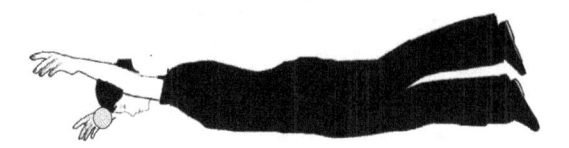

### Checklist
- ✓ Press the stomach and hips into the floor and tighten the buttocks muscles to protect the back
- ✓ Lift just one arm and leg at a time. Do not lift the other arm, leg, or head off the floor
- ✓ Use a pillow under the hips &/or towel roll under the forehead if needed
- ✓ Do not lift the arm and leg too high and strain the low back
- ✓ Use diaphragmatic breathing through the nose as much as possible
- ✓ Do not exercise to the point of strain or discomfort
- ✓ Remember the goal of yoga is to find that point where you are challenging yourself but not struggling

## Boat Pose

The next few poses are only shown lying down. If you are unable to do floor exercises skip ahead. Lie on your stomach with the hands down by your sides, palms facing the floor. Place your forehead or chin on the floor. To protect the neck it is not recommended that you turn your head to the side. If needed you can place a pillow under the hips or a towel roll under the forehead. Press your abdominal muscles and pelvic bones down into the floor and tighten the buttocks muscles. This will help to protect the back.

Bring your arms down by your sides with the palms facing the floor. Begin to lift your head, shoulders, chest, legs, and arms off the floor as high as you are able. Do not tilt the head back and compress the neck. Keep your gaze down at the floor. Reach your arms back and open the chest. Make sure you do not strain the low back. Only lift as high as you can without hurting your back. Hold for 5-10 deep belly breaths or to comfort.

*Lying flat*

*Lying with a pillow under hips & towel roll under head*

*Lift the head, shoulders, chest, legs and arms off the floor.*

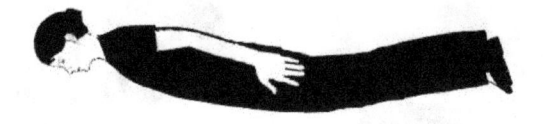

### Checklist
- ✓ Press the stomach and hips into the floor and tighten the buttocks muscles to protect the back
- ✓ Do not tilt the head back and compress the neck
- ✓ Use a pillow under the hips &/or towel roll under the forehead if needed
- ✓ Do not lift the arm and leg too high and strain the low back
- ✓ Use diaphragmatic breathing through the nose as much as possible
- ✓ Do not exercise to the point of strain or discomfort
- ✓ Remember the goal of yoga is to find that point where you are challenging yourself but not struggling

# Sphinx Pose

Lie on your stomach with the hands underneath your shoulders and palms facing the floor. Place your forehead or chin on the floor. To protect the neck it is not recommended that you turn your head to the side. If needed you can place a pillow under the hips or a towel roll under the forehead. Press your abdominal muscles and pelvic bones down into the floor and tighten the buttocks muscles. This will help to protect the back.

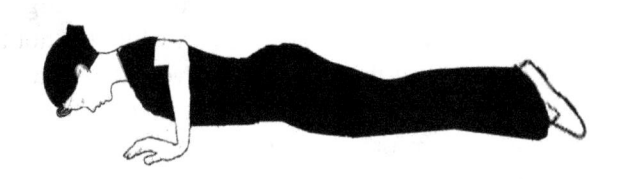

Using your low back muscles begin to lift your head, shoulders, and chest off the floor as high as you are able. Your arms can help support you but avoid using arm strength alone to lift up. Do not tilt the head back and compress the neck. Keep your gaze down at the floor. Lift as high as you can but do not strain the low back. If your back is sensitive place your elbows on the floor. Only lift as high as you can without hurting your back. Keep the shoulders down and away from the ears. Hold for 5-10 deep belly breaths or to comfort.

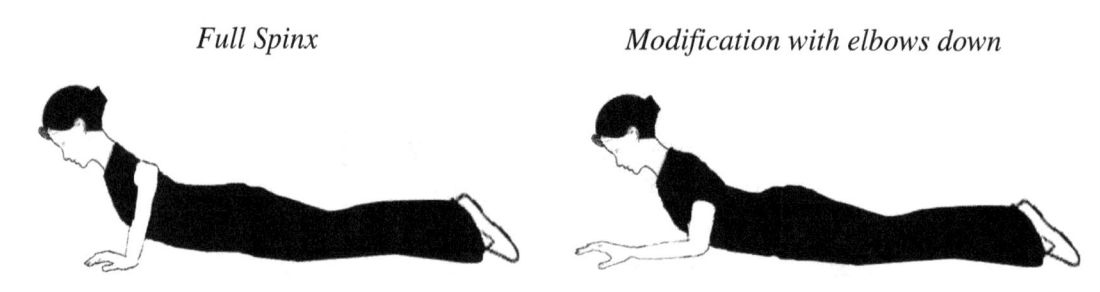

*Full Spinx*  *Modification with elbows down*

### Checklist
- Press the stomach and hips into the floor and tighten the buttocks muscles to protect the back
- Do not tilt the head back and compress the neck
- Use a pillow under the hips &/or towel roll under the forehead if needed
- Use the low back muscles, not the arms to lift you up
- Do not lift high and strain the low back
- Use diaphragmatic breathing through the nose as much as possible
- Do not exercise to the point of strain or discomfort
- Remember the goal of yoga is to find that point where you are challenging yourself but not struggling

## Cat and Dog Pose/Balancing Cat

Come up to hand and knees. Place your hands directly under your shoulders and your knees directly under your hips. If it bothers your wrists to be on your hands, you can either make fists with your hands or come down to your elbows.

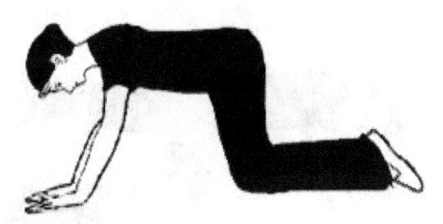

As you inhale begin to round the low back. Tuck your head in and look at your stomach.

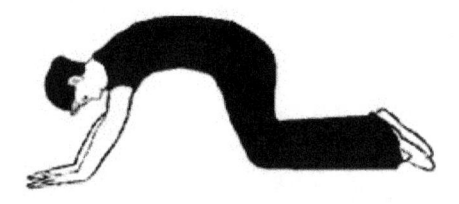

As you exhale come back to a neutral position. If it feels comfortable on your back you can let the belly move towards the floor and let the low back arch slightly. Do not bend the elbows. Keep the head and neck level. Do not tilt the head back and compress the neck. Move back and forth 8-12 times.

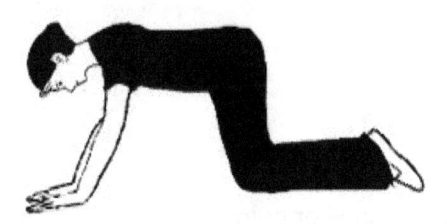

### Checklist
- ✓ Try to isolate the low back
- ✓ Do not bend the elbows during this exercise
- ✓ Use diaphragmatic breathing through the nose as much as possible
- ✓ Inhale as you round the back and exhale as you flatten the back
- ✓ Do not exercise to the point of strain or discomfort
- ✓ Remember the goal of yoga is to find that point where you are challenging yourself but not struggling

## Balancing Cat

Next, lift your right arm and left leg off the floor and balance. The right elbow should be by your ear. Do not let the right arm drift off to the side. Keep your left knee as straight as you can. Hold for 5-10 deep belly breaths or to comfort. Repeat with the left arm and right leg.

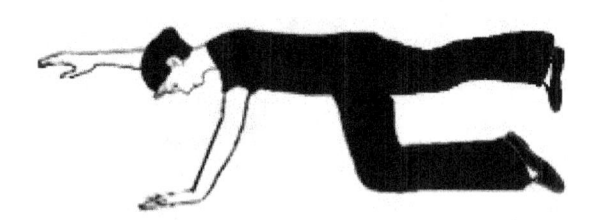

Checklist
- ✓ Make fists with your hands or come down to your elbows if your wrists are sensitive
- ✓ Keep the elbows straight throughout this movement
- ✓ Use diaphragmatic breathing through the nose as much as possible
- ✓ Do not exercise to the point of strain or discomfort
- ✓ Remember the goal of yoga is to find that point where you are challenging yourself but not struggling

## Child Pose

The last few postures have focused on arching the low back and opening the chest. It is always good to balance your practice by moving the body in opposing ways. Child pose will help to relax the low back and provides a counter stretch for the back.

Come up to hands and knees. Let the hips drop back and bring them as close to your heels as you can. Let the head relax on the floor. The object of this pose is to let your body relax. Avoid holding this posture with your head off of the floor.

If your knees are sensitive you can place a pillow between the heels and buttocks to reduce the bend in the knees. If your head will not comfortably rest on the floor place a pillow under the forehead so the neck can relax. Hold for 5-10 deep belly breaths or to comfort.

*Bring the hips to the heels and the head to the floor.*

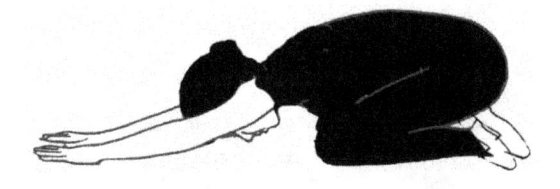

Modify by placing a pillow between the heels and hips &/or a pillow under the head.

Checklist
- ✓ Use a pillow under the buttocks &/or forehead if needed
- ✓ To support the neck your head should be touching the floor or a pillow
- ✓ Use diaphragmatic breathing through the nose as much as possible
- ✓ Do not exercise to the point of strain or discomfort
- ✓ Remember the goal of yoga is to find that point where you are challenging yourself but not struggling

## Strap Stretches

For the following 3 stretches you can use a yoga strap or a long sheet or towel. The goal of the strap is to assist you in getting a deeper stretch. However, it is important to not pull hard with the strap as this can cause the muscles to tighten up instead of relax and stretch. Do all of the stretches on one leg first and then switch legs.

## Hamstring Stretch

Keeping the low back tight against the floor bring your right knee towards your chest. Wrap the towel or strap under the ball of the right foot. Then straighten the leg, flex the foot, and press the heel up towards the ceiling. Straighten the leg as much as you can but do not lock the knee. If this bothers your low back you can also leave a soft bend in the knee. Hold the ends of the towel or strap with your hands. Make sure your head stays on the floor or pillow. Do not hold the head off the floor as this strains the neck. Let the elbows come to the floor to fully relax the shoulders. If the back or hips are sensitive keep the left knee bent with the foot on the floor. For a deeper stretch extend the left leg out straight on the floor. Hold for five to ten deep belly breaths or for as long as is comfortable.

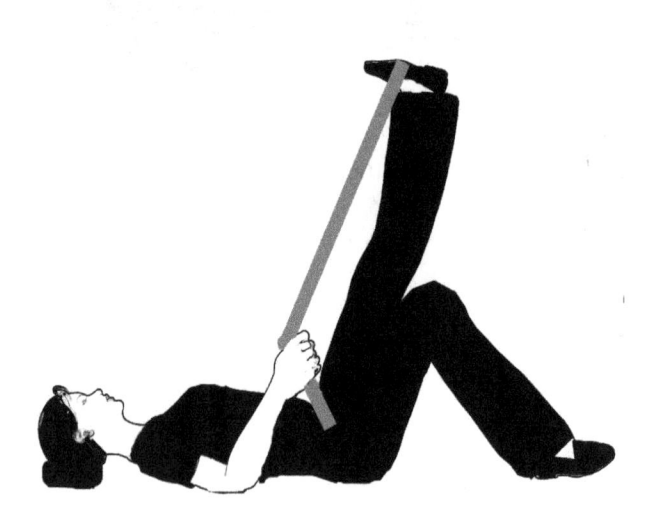

## Seated Version

Sit up against the back of the chair. Wrap the strap or towel around the ball of the right foot. Extend your right leg forward and pull the toes towards you. Keep the back straight and shoulders down away from the ears.

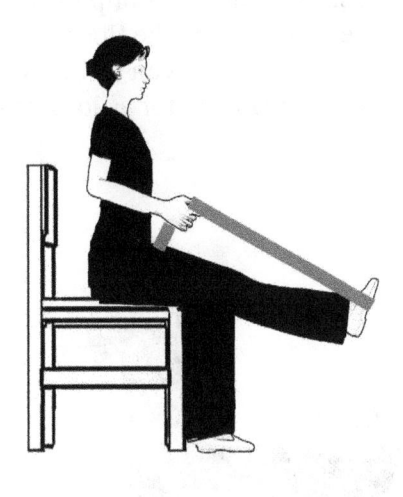

### Checklist
- ✓ Make sure you keep your head and chin level and your head on the floor or pillow
- ✓ Make sure you keep the low back in contact with the floor
- ✓ The knee can be straight or have a soft bend, do not lock the knee
- ✓ Use diaphragmatic breathing through the nose as much as possible
- ✓ Hold for five to ten deep belly breaths
- ✓ Do not exercise to the point of strain or discomfort
- ✓ To support the neck your head should be touching the floor or a pillow
- ✓ Use diaphragmatic breathing through the nose as much as possible
- ✓ Do not exercise to the point of strain or discomfort
- ✓ Remember the goal of yoga is to find that point where you are challenging yourself but not struggling

## Inner Thigh Stretch

Keep the low back tight against the floor and place both ends of the strap in your right hand. Let the leg drop out to the right to stretch the inner thigh. If comfortable let the left hip roll off the floor and let the right foot come as close to the floor as possible. If the back is sensitive remain in a pelvic tilt and keep the right foot up off the floor. Straighten the right leg as much as you can but do not lock the knee. Make sure your head stays on the floor or pillow. Do not hold the head off the floor as this strains the neck. Let the right elbow come to the floor. Stretch the left arm out to the side in a "T" position with the palm facing up. The left knee can be bent or straight depending on your hips and back. Hold for five to ten deep belly breaths or for as long as is comfortable.

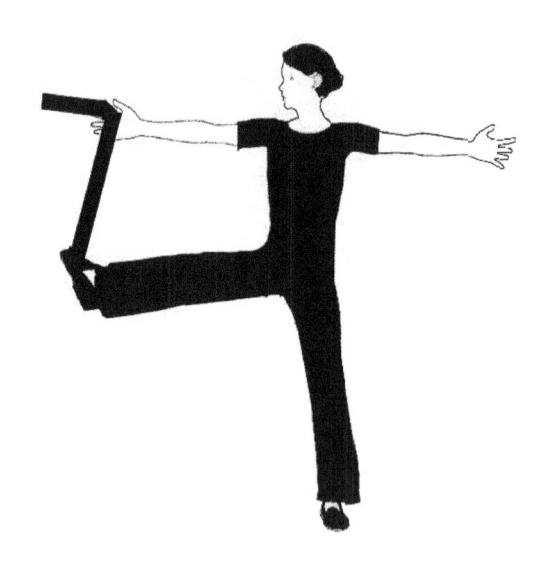

## Seated Version

Sit against the back of the chair. Wrap the strap or towel around the ball of the right foot. Turn the right leg out slightly and carry it out to the side without twisting the hips. Keep the back straight and shoulders down away from the ears.

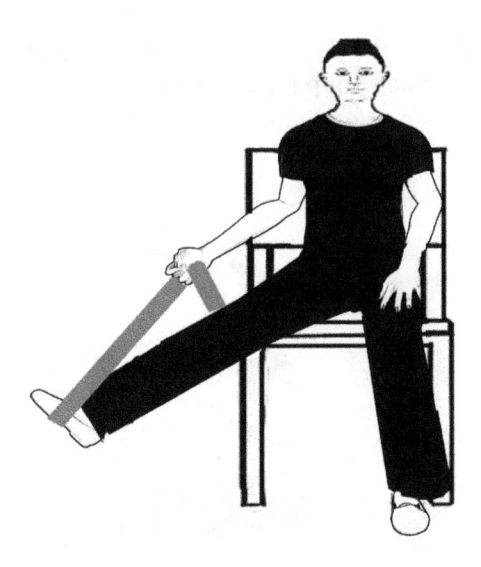

### Checklist
- ✓ Make sure you keep your head and chin level and your head on the floor or pillow
- ✓ Make sure you keep the low back in contact with the floor
- ✓ The knee can be straight or have a soft bend, do not lock the knee
- ✓ Use diaphragmatic breathing through the nose as much as possible
- ✓ Hold for five to ten deep belly breaths
- ✓ Do not exercise to the point of strain or discomfort
- ✓ Use diaphragmatic breathing through the nose as much as possible
- ✓ Do not exercise to the point of strain or discomfort
- ✓ Remember the goal of yoga is to find that point where you are challenging yourself but not struggling

## Outer Hip Stretch

Bring the leg back up to center and place both ends of the strap in your left hand. Bring the right leg across the body to stretch the outer hip and back. If comfortable let the right hip roll off the floor and let the right foot come as close to the floor as possible. If the back is sensitive remain in a pelvic tilt and keep the right foot up off the floor. Straighten the right leg as much as you can but do not lock the knee. Make sure your head stays on the floor or pillow. Do not hold the head off the floor as this strains the neck. Let the left elbow come to the floor. Stretch the right arm out to the side in a "T" position with the palm facing up. The left knee can stay bent or straight depending on your hips and back. Hold for five to ten deep belly breaths or for as long as is comfortable.

Use caution with this stretch if you have had a hip replacement or have compression fractures in the back. Check with your health care provider about the appropriateness of this stretch. If in doubt follow the instructions for the seated modification.

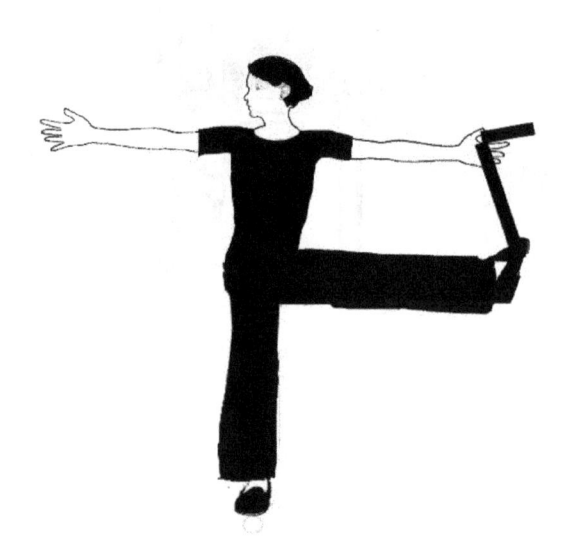

## Seated Version

You may need to follow the modification if you have had a hip replacement so check with your physician about the appropriateness of this exercise. Sit up straight. For this stretch you may wish to sit against the back of the chair to support your back. Bring your right ankle bone up to the left knee. Let the right knee drop out to the side as much as possible. Make sure that you are not just crossing the legs. It should be your right ankle bone on your left knee, not your right knee. If modifying cross your right ankle over your left ankle and let the right knee fall out to the side as much as possible. Hold for 5-10 deep belly breaths, or to comfort. Repeat with the left leg.

Hip Stretch       Modification

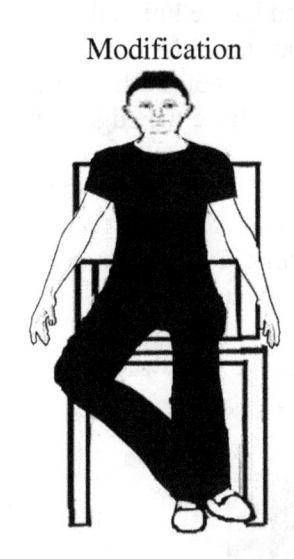

### Checklist
- ✓ Sit up straight
- ✓ Use diaphragmatic breathing through the nose as much as possible
- ✓ Hold for five to ten deep belly breaths
- ✓ Do the modified version if you have had a hip replacement
- ✓ Do not exercise to the point of strain or discomfort
- ✓ To support the neck your head should be touching the floor or a pillow
- ✓ Use diaphragmatic breathing through the nose as much as possible
- ✓ Do not exercise to the point of strain or discomfort
- ✓ Remember the goal of yoga is to find that point where you are challenging yourself but not struggling

## Bound Angle

The goal of this posture is to allow the body to completely relax. This posture helps to open the shoulders and chest. You will need a yoga bolster or you can use a couch cushion or a pile of blankets and a few pillows.

If your neck is sensitive you can use the cushion the long way so that your head is supported. If your neck does not bother you, use the cushion the short way so that your neck and head come off the end of the cushion.

To get into this posture, sit up straight and place the bolster behind you, do not sit on it. Bring the soles of your feet together and let the knees drop out to the side. Place a pillow underneath each knee. The purpose of this posture is to let the whole body completely relax, so let the pillows support your knees if they do not reach the floor. Then, lie down over the cushion. If you are using the cushion the short way have the edge of it come just underneath your armpits so your shoulders are off the cushion.

The closer the heels are to the body the deeper the stretch, so adjust your heels accordingly. To support the neck you can also place a pillow or rolled up towel underneath the neck. Hold this posture for as long as feels comfortable. Take deep belly breaths into the chest and shoulders and let your body sink and rest into the cushions.

Using the bolster the long way         Using the bolster the short way

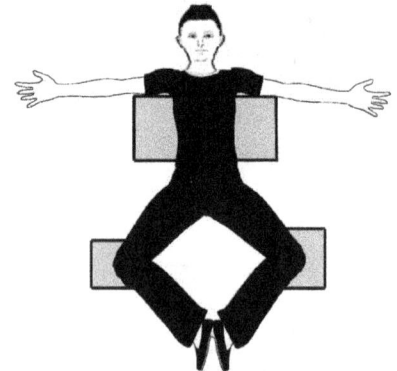

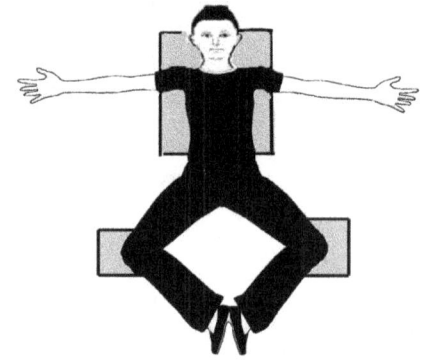

### Checklist
- ✓ Make sure your neck is supported and do not let the head tip back
- ✓ Use pillows to support the knees if they do not reach the floor to allow your leg muscles to fully relax
- ✓ Use diaphragmatic breathing through the nose as much as possible
- ✓ Do not exercise to the point of strain or discomfort
- ✓ Remember the goal of yoga is to find that point where you are challenging yourself but not struggling

# T'ai Chi

Tai chi is a gentle low-impact traditional Chinese form of exercise that combines meditation and movement to improve and maintain health. It combines deep breathing with movements that flow slowly and smoothly from one to the other. The practice of Tai chi can help to enhance balance and body awareness and aid in making daily activities such as dressing walking, climbing, bending, and lifting easier.

Some of the principals of Tai chi are:

1) Energy (called chi) flows through the body along "energy pathways" called meridians. Illness may occur if the flow of chi is blocked or unbalanced at any point on these pathways. Tai chi is practiced to increase a person's chi energy and improve health through gentle, graceful, repeated movements.

2) Separate yin and yang. Nature including the body, consists of opposing forces called yin and yang and good health results when these forces are in balance. Tai chi movements are done in an attempt to help restore the body's balance of yin and yang. For example, if all of your weight is in your left leg then the left leg is yang and the unweighted right leg is yin. The goal is to become aware of this process.

3) Relaxation. The body should remain relaxed during Tai chi movements. The attention should be on continuously releasing tension especially in the neck, wrists, shoulders, and knees.

4) Turn from the waist. Eyes, nose and navel should turn as one unit.

5) The body is upright. As with all of the exercises in this book use good posture. The head remains upright. Think about lifting the crown of the head to the ceiling (without lifting the chin) or being suspended from the ceiling by a string.

6) Tai chi has been promoted for improved health, memory, concentration, digestion, balance and flexibility. It may also aid in improving conditions such as anxiety, depression, and age-related declines in mental function. Studies have found that people who practice Tai chi are not as fearful of activity and are more confident when moving about. Tai chi includes movements that strengthen the legs. The exercises also provide an opportunity to explore where your center of gravity is, thereby exploring your balance. With practice you learn how to move your center of gravity. This can help you to become more aware of when you are getting unsteady and when you are not. As you begin to get things mapped out in your head, you gain more confidence, become more precise in your reactions, and more conscious of when you may be putting yourself at risk for a fall.

T'ai Chi has been promoted for improved health, memory, concentration, digestion, balance and flexibility. It may also aid in improving conditions such as anxiety, depression, and age-related declines in mental function. Studies have found that people who practice T'ai Chi are not as fearful of activity and are more confident when moving about.

The exercises are shown in standing and seated versions try to do as much as you can standing to help improve your balance and use the seated versions on days when you feel unable to stand.

# T'ai Chi Movements

## Pressing Energy Down

Check your posture before you begin. Shoulders should be back and down and over the hips. Knees should remain slightly bent. Tuck in the chin and think about pushing the crown of the head up to the ceiling without lifting your chin. The abdominal muscles are lightly pulled in, but not so much that it restricts your breathing.

Stand with the feet shoulder to hip width apart and knees slightly bent. Arms are down by your side with the palms facing forward. Raise your arms to shoulder height with the palms facing the ceiling.

Next, turn the hands so the palms face the floor, and slightly bend the elbows and wrists. Bring the arms back down to your side. Practice deep belly breathing but do not try to coordinate your breath with the movement. Repeat eight to twelve times.

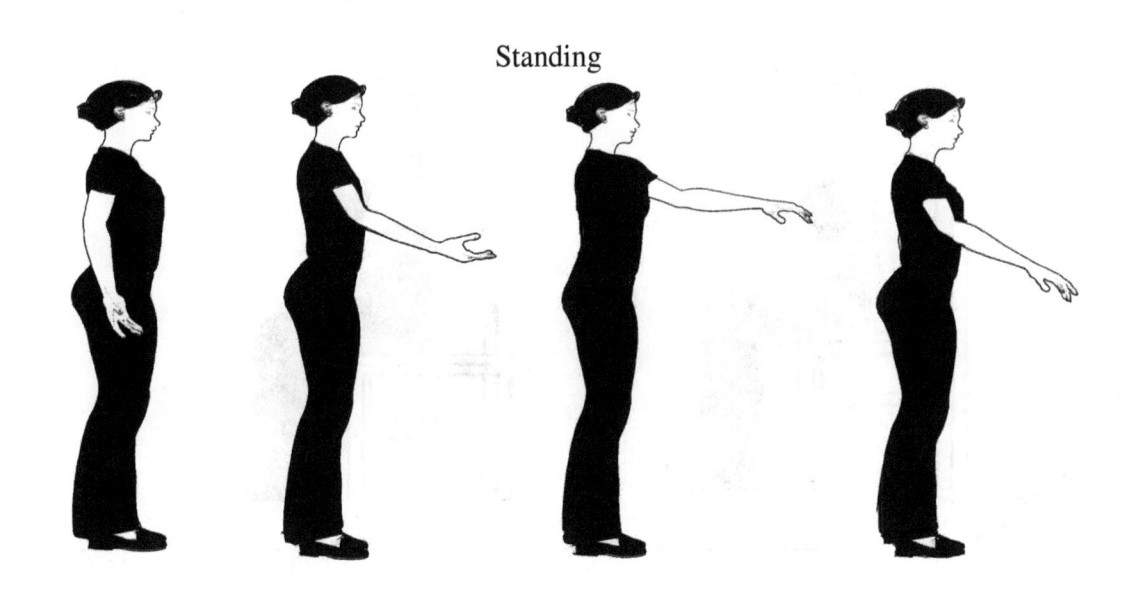

Standing

Seated

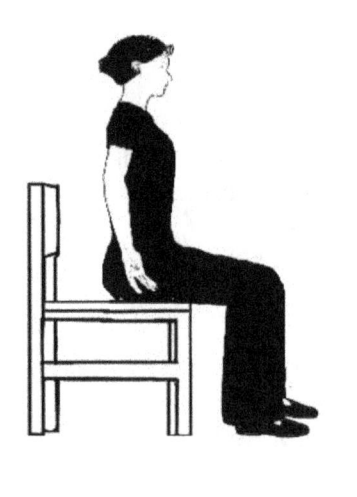

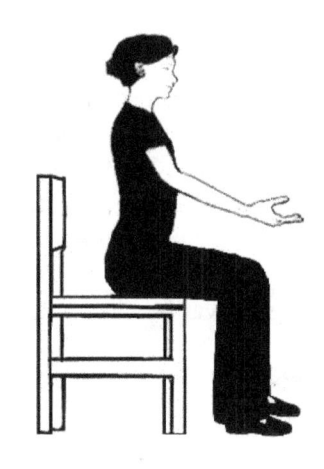

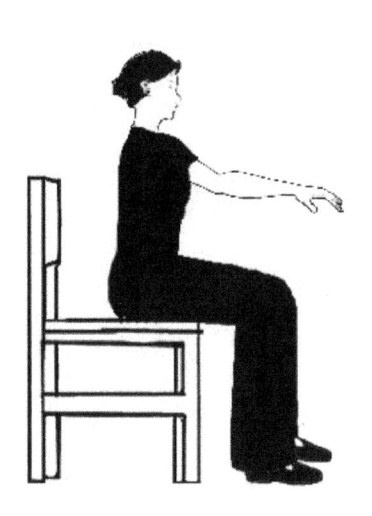

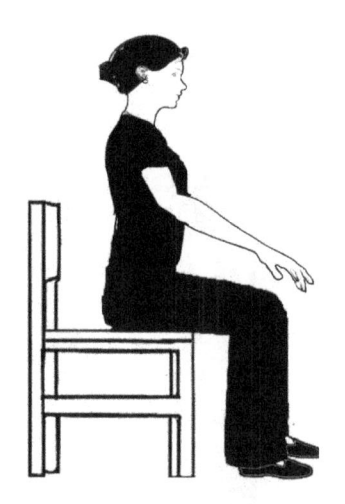

### Checklist
- Stand or sit up straight
- Keep the shoulders down away from the ears
- Keep the natural curve in the low back
- Keep the knees, elbows and wrists soft and slightly bent
- Use diaphragmatic breathing through the nose as much as possible
- In traditional T'ai Chi practice the eyes always remain open - however, to further challenge your balance, you can try closing the eyes during this exercise
- Do not exercise to the point of strain or discomfort

## Spreading The Eagle's Wings

Check your posture before you begin. Shoulders should be back and down and over the hips. Knees should remain slightly bent. Tuck in the chin and think about pushing the crown of the head up to the ceiling without lifting your chin. The abdominal muscles are lightly pulled in, but not so much that it restricts your breathing.

Stand with your feet hip width apart and knees slightly bent. Your hands are in front of the body with the palms facing each other. Lift your arms in front of the body (as if you were hugging a tree) and then into a circle overhead. With the arms overhead, turn the palms to face away from each other. Bend the elbows and wrists. Bring the arms back down to your side. Repeat 8-12 times. Practice deep belly breathing. Allow your breath to be slow and deep throughout the movement.

Standing

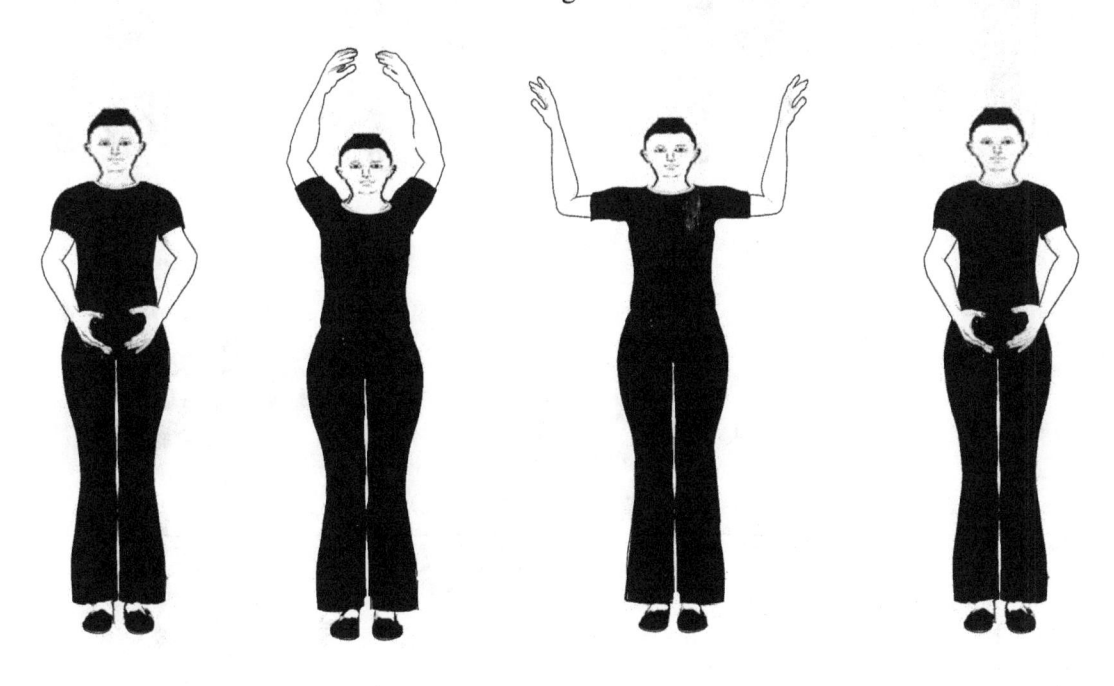

Seated

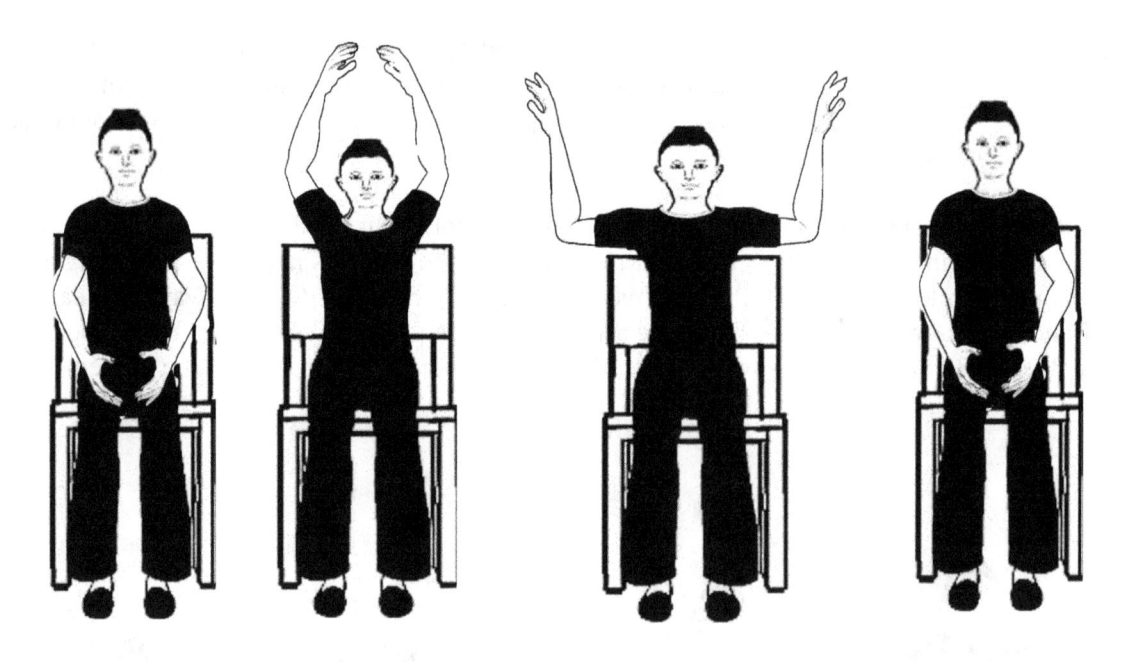

### Checklist
- Stand or sit up straight
- Keep the shoulders down away from the ears
- Keep the natural curve in the low back
- Keep the knees, elbows and wrists soft and slightly bent
- Use diaphragmatic breathing through the nose as much as possible
- In traditional T'ai Chi practice the eyes always remain open - however, to further challenge your balance, you can try closing the eyes during this exercise
- Do not exercise to the point of strain or discomfort

## Gathering Energy

Check your posture before you begin. Shoulders should be back and down and over the hips. Knees should remain slightly bent. Tuck in the chin and think about pushing the crown of the head up to the ceiling without lifting your chin. The abdominal muscles are lightly pulled in, but not so much that it restricts your breathing.

Stand with feet shoulder to hip width apart and keep your knees slightly bent. Arms are by your sides with the arms and shoulders rotated out and the palms facing away from you. Raise the arms shoulder height with the palms facing the ceiling. Bring the palms towards each other at forehead height, forming a triangle with the arms. With the palms facing down, press the hands towards the floor.

Finish by bringing the arms back to your side. Repeat eight to twelve times. Allow your breath to be slow and deep throughout the movement, but do not try to coordinate your breath with the movement.

Standing

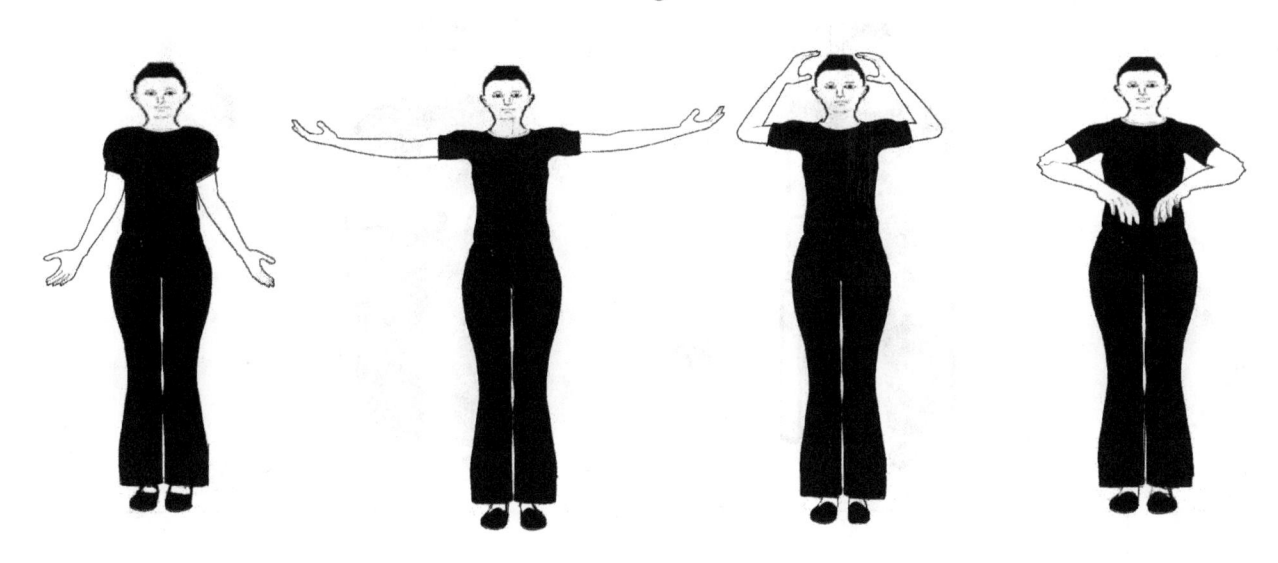

Seated

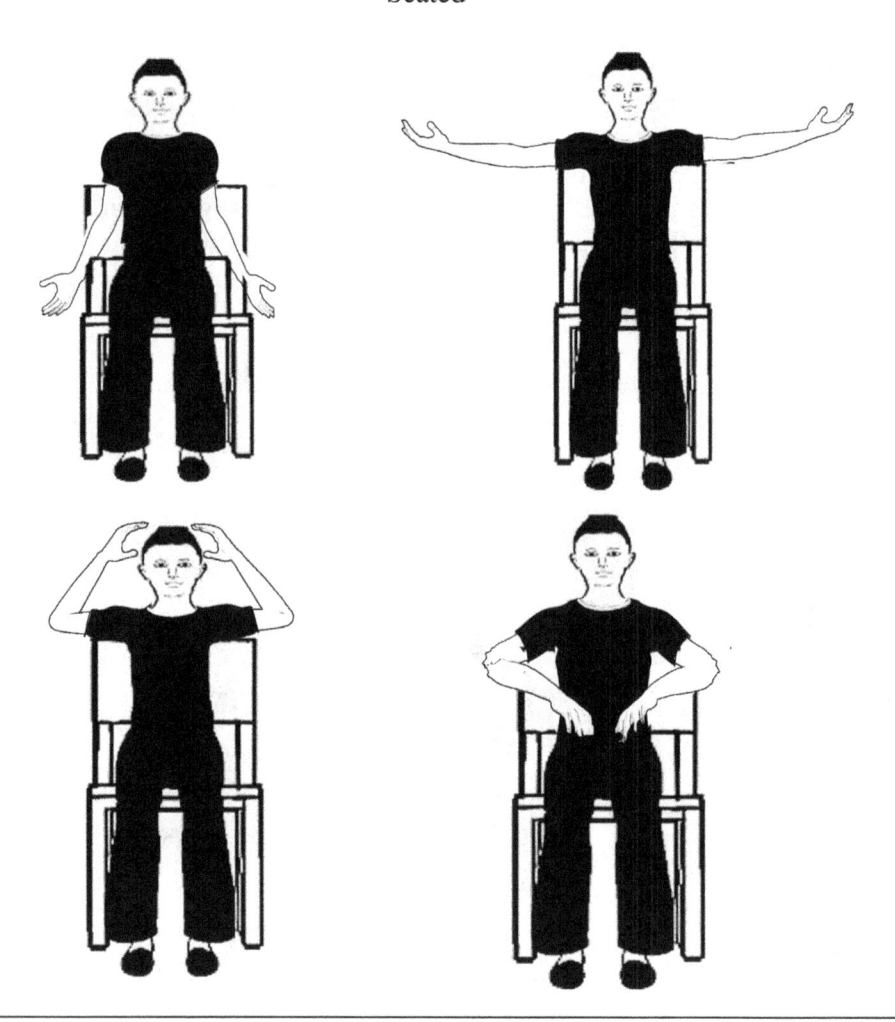

### Checklist
- Stand or sit up straight
- Keep the shoulders down away from the ears
- Keep the natural curve in the low back
- Keep the knees, elbows and wrists soft and slightly bent
- Use diaphragmatic breathing through the nose as much as possible
- In traditional T'ai Chi practice the eyes always remain open - however, to further challenge your balance, you can try closing the eyes during this exercise
- Do not exercise to the point of strain or discomfort

## Waist Twists

Check your posture before you begin. Shoulders should be back and down and over the hips. Knees should remain slightly bent. Tuck in the chin and think about pushing the crown of the head up to the ceiling without lifting your chin. The abdominal muscles are lightly pulled in, but not so much that it restricts your breathing.

If you have any back sensitivities use caution with this movement. Check with your health care provider if you have any concerns about the appropriateness of twisting motions.

Stand with the feet shoulder to hip width apart and knees slightly bent. Turning at the waist, press the right arm forward and your left arm straight behind you. Flex the hands and press through the palms to fully stretch the wrists and shoulders. Look back at your left hand. *Do not turn at the knees. The knees point straight ahead as you turn at the waist.* Come back to the center. Repeat on the left. Repeat 8-12 times to each side. Allow your breath to be slow and deep throughout the movement, but do not try to coordinate your breath with the movement.

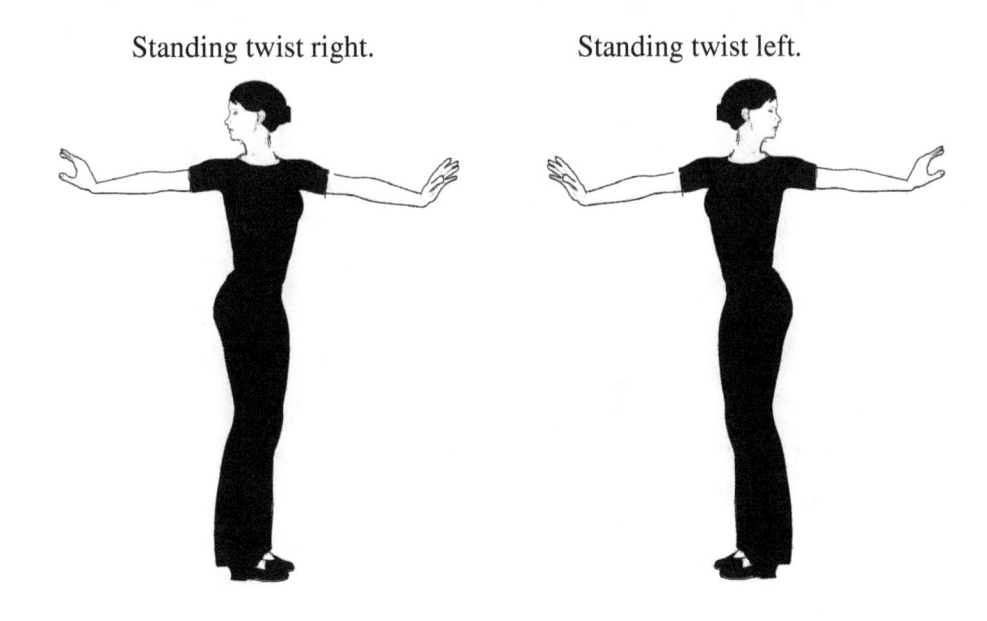

Standing twist right.

Standing twist left.

Seated twist right.  Seated twist left.

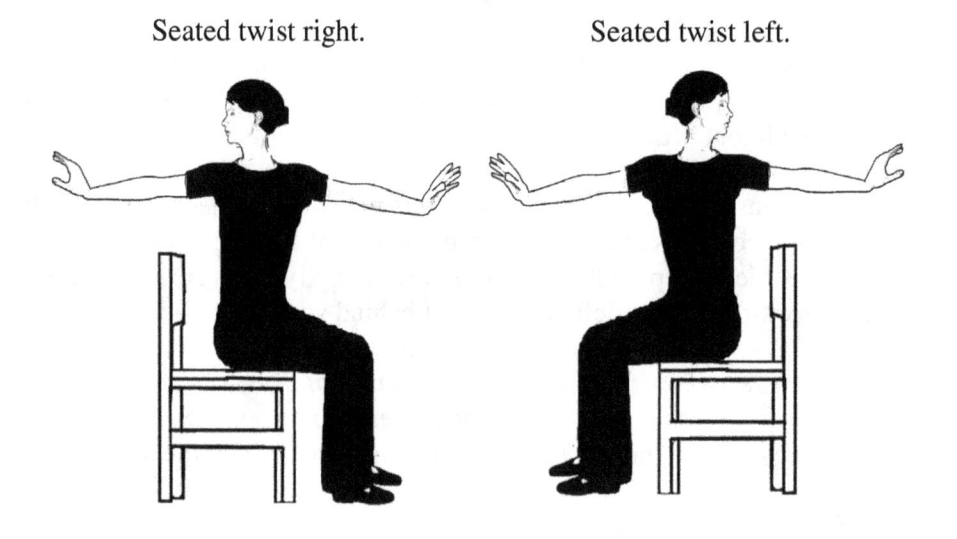

| Checklist |
|---|
| ✓ Stand or sit up straight |
| ✓ Keep the shoulders down away from the ears |
| ✓ Keep the natural curve in the low back |
| ✓ Keep the knees, elbows and wrists soft and slightly bent |
| ✓ Twist at the waist and keep the knees pointed forward |
| ✓ Use diaphragmatic breathing through the nose as much as possible |
| ✓ To further challenge your balance, you can try closing the eyes during this exercise |
| ✓ Do not exercise to the point of strain or discomfort |

## Side Bends

Check your posture before you begin. Shoulders should be back and down and over the hips. Knees should remain slightly bent. Tuck in the chin and think about pushing the crown of the head up to the ceiling without lifting your chin. The abdominal muscles are lightly pulled in, but not so much that it restricts your breathing.

Stand with the feet hip width apart and knees slightly bent. Bend to the right and press the right palm down towards the knee and the left palm up to the ceiling. Flex the hands and press through the palms to fully stretch the wrists and shoulders. Look up at your top hand. *Do not twist as you bend; the shoulders and the hips stay facing straight ahead. Pretend you are between two panes of glass and can only bend to the side.* Come back to the center. Repeat to the left. Repeat 8-12 times to each side. Allow your breath to be slow and deep throughout the movement, but do not try to coordinate your breath with the movement.

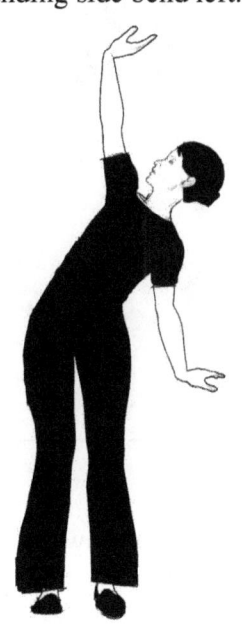

Standing side bend right.

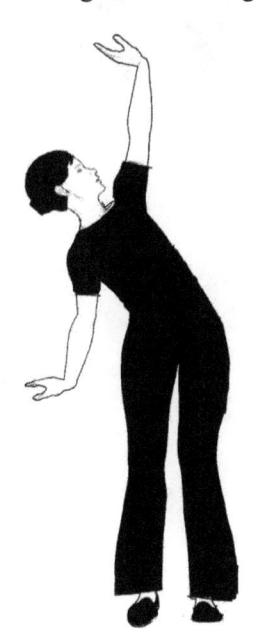

Standing side bend left.

Seated side bend right.　　　　Seated side bend left.

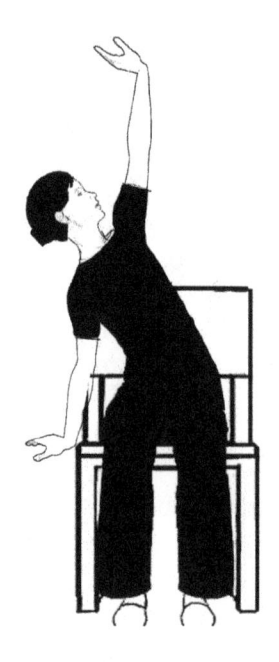

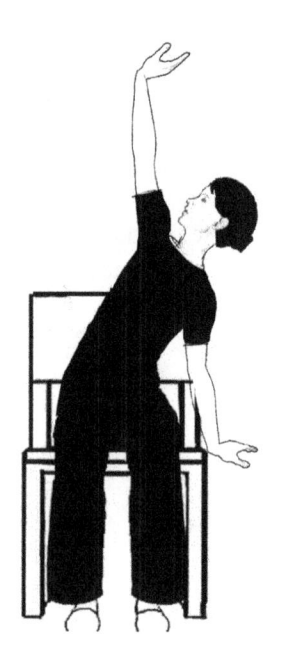

### Checklist
- ✓ Stand or sit up straight
- ✓ Keep the shoulders down away from the ears
- ✓ Keep the natural curve in the low back
- ✓ Keep the knees, elbows and wrists soft and slightly bent
- ✓ Just bend to the side without twisting
- ✓ Use diaphragmatic breathing through the nose as much as possible
- ✓ To further challenge your balance, you can try closing the eyes during this exercise
- ✓ Do not exercise to the point of strain or discomfort

## Tai chi Walk

This is meant to be a traveling movement and is only shown standing. If your balance is challenged you can do this exercise in a hallway using your hands against the wall for support or walk along next to a counter top.

Check your posture before you begin. Shoulders should be back and down and over the hips. Knees should remain slightly bent. Tuck in the chin and think about pushing the crown of the head up to the ceiling without lifting your chin. The abdominal muscles are lightly pulled in, but not so much that it restricts your breathing.

Bend the right knee lifting the right foot off of the floor. Bend the elbows and lift the lower arms up with the palms facing the ceiling. Place the right heel on the floor as the palms turn and push forward. Lower the right toes and lunge forward as the arms straighten out to the front. Step the left foot up to the right foot as the arms lower to your side. Repeat left foot.

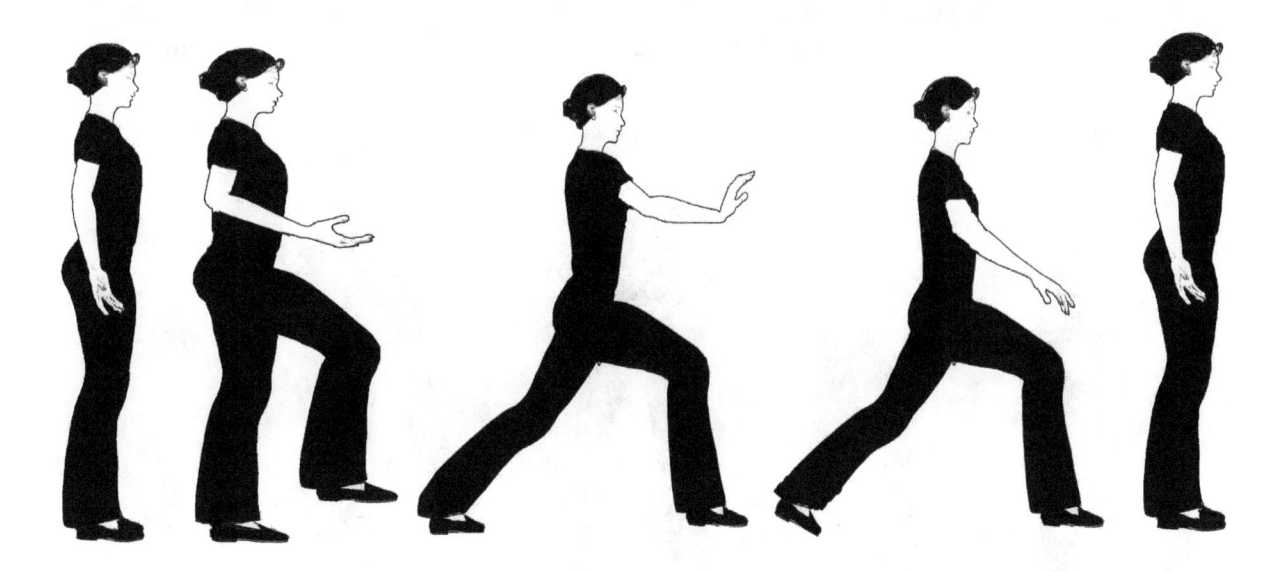

| Checklist |
|---|
| ✓ Stand up straight |
| ✓ Keep the shoulders down away from the ears |
| ✓ Keep the natural curve in the low back |
| ✓ Keep the knees, elbows and wrists soft and slightly bent |
| ✓ Take smaller steps or hold onto a counter top or wall if balance is difficult |
| ✓ Use diaphragmatic breathing through the nose as much as possible |
| ✓ Do not exercise to the point of strain or discomfort |

## Chasing Clouds

This is a traveling movement to help improve balance and is only shown standing. If you find your balance is challenged you can do the leg movements while holding onto a counter or table.

Check your posture before you begin. Shoulders should be back and down and over the hips. Knees should remain slightly bent. Tuck in the chin and think about pushing the crown of the head up to the ceiling without lifting your chin. The abdominal muscles are lightly pulled in, but not so much that it restricts your breathing.

Hands are at your right side with the left hand on top like you are holding a small ball. Look to the right. Bend your left knee and pick up your left foot as high as you can keeping your balance. Step out to the left. Land in a squat position with *equal weight on both feet.* Turn the hands so that the right hand is on top. Keep the legs still as you carry the pretend ball to the center. Next, step the right foot to the left as you bring the hands and the pretend ball to your left side. Look to your left. Then bring the hands back to the right. Change so the left hand is on top again, and you are looking right. Repeat three more times to the left. Reverse the directions, traveling four times right. Take slow deep breaths but do not try to coordinate your breath with the movement.

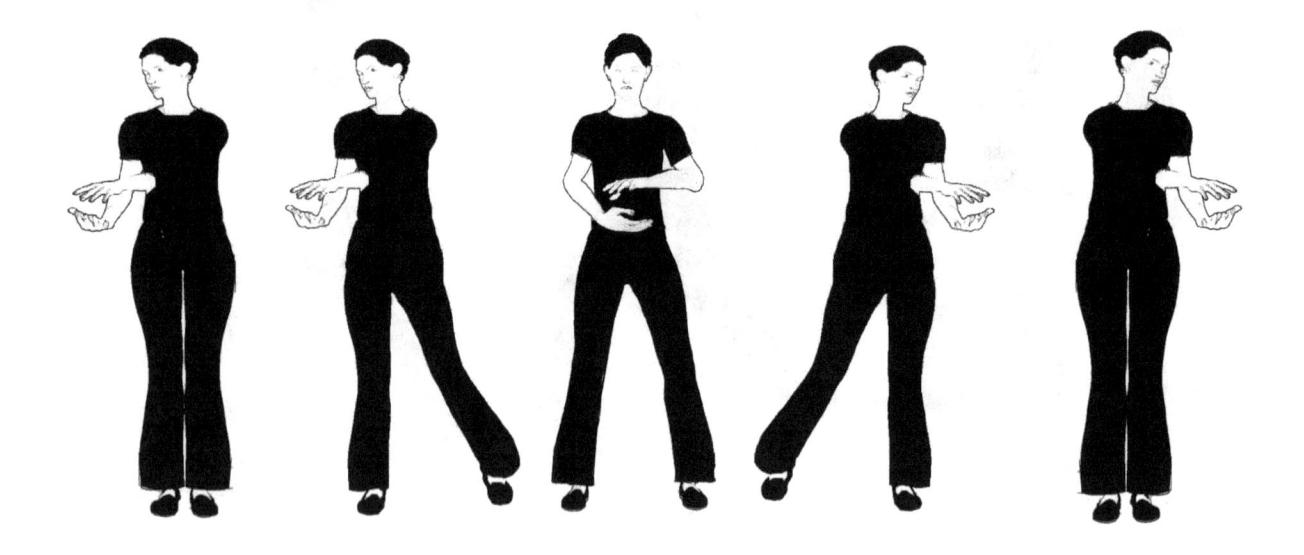

### Checklist
- ✓ Stand or sit up straight
- ✓ Keep the shoulders down away from the ears
- ✓ Keep the knees, elbows and wrists soft and slightly bent
- ✓ Use diaphragmatic breathing through the nose as much as possible
- ✓ Do not exercise to the point of strain or discomfort

# Tandem Walking

Another exercise that is helpful for balance is called Tandem Walking. This exercise is not a traditional tai chi movement but it is very good for improving balance. It involves slowly walking forward and backward with the feet tight together. If you find this challenging you can do this exercise walking down a hallway with your hands on the walls or walk along with one hand on a counter top.

Stand up straight with the left foot in front of the right. Next, step the right foot in front of the left with the heel flexed and the heel of the front foot touching the toe of the back foot. Then repeat putting the left foot forward so the left heel and right toes are touching. To get the most from this exercise make sure the heel and toes touch and do not separate the feet. Take a few steps forward. Take slow deep breaths but do not try to coordinate your breath with the movement.

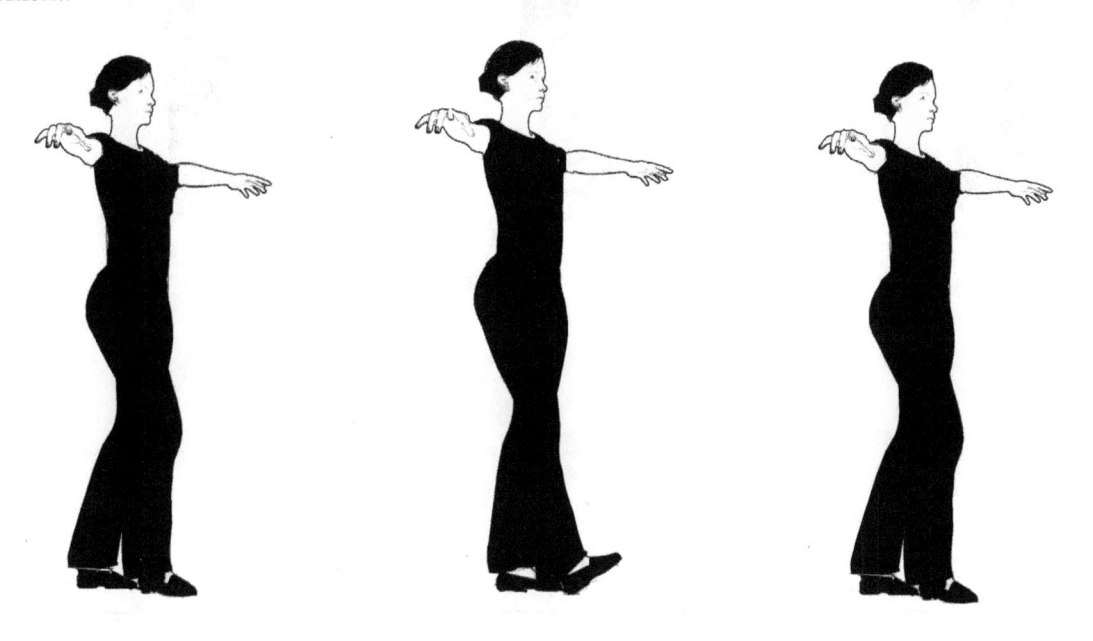

Then repeat going backwards. Place the right foot behind the left with the right toes touching the left heel. Then reach the left foot back touching the left toe and right heel. Take a few steps backwards. Take slow deep breaths but do not try to coordinate your breath with the movement.

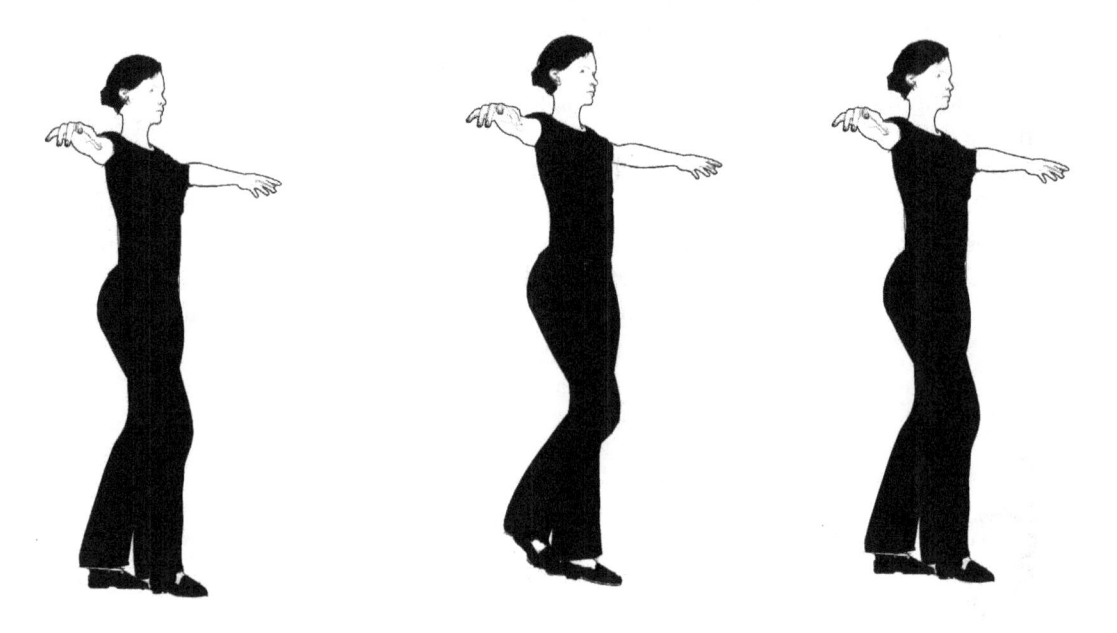

| Checklist |
|---|
| ✓ Stand up straight |
| ✓ Keep the shoulders down away from the ears |
| ✓ Keep the natural curve in the low back |
| ✓ Go slowly and work on maintaining balance the entire time |
| ✓ Use diaphragmatic breathing through the nose as much as possible |
| ✓ Do not exercise to the point of strain or discomfort |

## Summary

A yoga and T'ai chi practice can be a great addition to an aerobic and strength training routine. Regular stretching is essential to help those with osteoporosis maintain range of motion and the body awareness gained through yoga and T'ai chi, will help to reduce the risk of falls.

For best results you can vary your routine by performing aerobics and strength training exercises three times a week and practice yoga or T'ai chi postures on two or three alternate days. This will give you a well rounded program to help manage all of your symptoms.

Another component of yoga is learning to manage stress. The next chapter will address how stress can affect your body and it also outlines several techniques you can try to help reduce tension.

# Chapter 6
## Relaxation Techniques and Stress Management.

*Happiness is not found at the end of the road, it is experienced along the way. So take not for granted each moment of your life and you will find a reason to be happy each day. Don't worry so much about tomorrow that you forget to live today."*

### *What is stress*

Stress is not a disease but rather a normal part of everyone's life. Stress is any event that an organism must adapt to, and it does not necessarily have a negative or positive correlation. Stress results from situations that require one to change and/or adjust behaviorally and such changes can be positive or negative. Examples of stress include the body responding to the pressures of gravity, physiological adaptations to an exercise regimen, or changes to one's way of life. Stress can include feelings of mental or emotional strain, suspense, anxiety, fear, worry, tension, excitement, or a general feeling of uneasiness or dread in response to a real or imagined threat. Any sort of change can make you feel stressed, even good change. It's not just the change or event itself that matters, but how you react to it. Therefore the word stress does not always need to be associated with a negative event. What may be stressful is different for each person. For example, although one person may not feel stressed about retiring from work, another person may. Getting married is a joyous event. It is also stressful for many. Having to adjust to an illness or financial changes can be stressful. In life, we have to constantly adjust to change. Exposure to stress becomes a issue when the stressor is perceived as something to which one can not adapt to, control, or when an individual believes that he or she is unable to cope with the situation.

### *What happens to the body when we feel stressed*

Stress is caused by the body's natural instinct to defend itself. In the case of emergencies such as getting out of the way of a speeding car this instinct is good, but it can cause physical symptoms if it goes on for too long, such as in response to life's daily challenges and changes. Stress evokes the fight-or-flight response. The fight-or-flight response is characterized by increased metabolism, heart rate, breathing, and blood pressure all of which prepare us to run or to fight, and this can lead to a number of stress-related symptoms.

In order for the above reactions to occur, the various systems of the body must signal and communicate with one another. The body-mind accomplishes this communication through the use of messenger molecules controlled by various systems of the body. These messenger molecules help to send and receive signals that activate both voluntary and involuntary actions. Some of the systems of the body include the nervous system, the neuropeptide system, the immune system, and the endocrine system.

*The Nervous System*

This system is comprised of the central nervous system (CNS) and the peripheral nervous system. The peripheral system connects the CNS to sensory receptors and motor neurons allowing the CNS to communicate with the muscles and glands. The peripheral nervous system is further divided into the autonomic nervous system which includes the sympathetic nervous system and the parasympathetic nervous system.

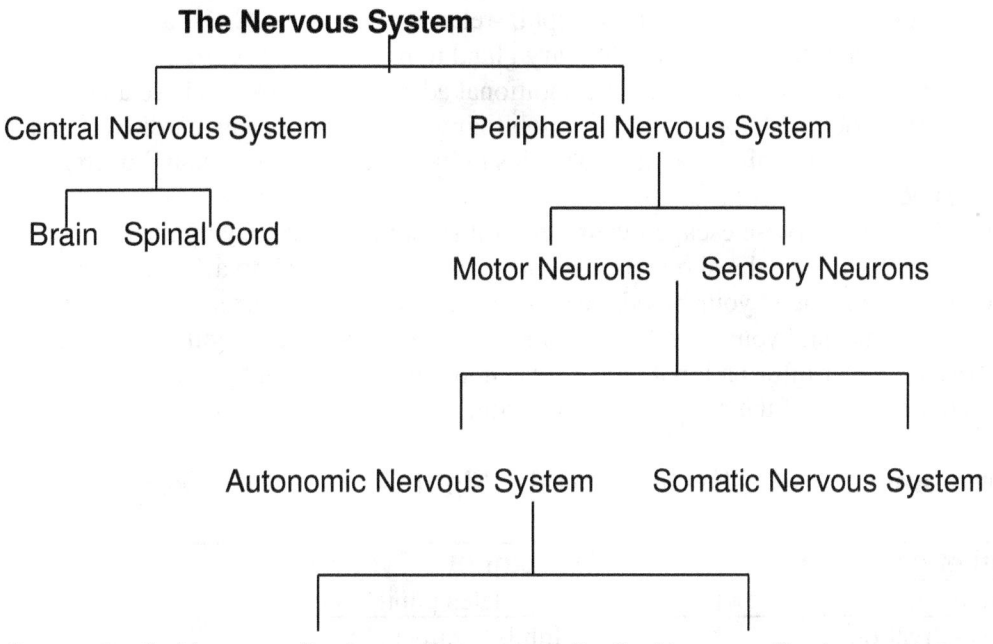

**The Nervous System**
- Central Nervous System
  - Brain
  - Spinal Cord
- Peripheral Nervous System
  - Motor Neurons
  - Sensory Neurons
    - Autonomic Nervous System
      - Sympathetic Nervous System
      - Parasympathetic Nervous System
    - Somatic Nervous System

*What is the stress response*

Research suggests that constant exposure to even mild stress over a prolonged period of time may have a detrimental effect on the body. These studies also suggest that stress management could potentially play a role in the management and treatment of many common ailments. In cases where there is a threat to our survival or physical well being the stress response is activated as needed, but then it is deactivated when the threat has passed. However, problems occur when the stress response is not deactivated. The stress response can become a constant occurrence in our daily life - during an argument, being stuck in traffic, experiencing financial difficulties, or when facing a chronic illness. While these situations may not be life threatening, whenever the body-mind senses that we are worried or "stressed" the fight or flight response is stimulated. If we constantly feel the pressures of such situations during daily life, then our body-mind is in a constant state of arousal.

The stress response occurs when an individual is exposed to a perceived danger. Then, in less then a second, the sympathetic nervous system (SNS) is signaled to release catecholamines such as epinephrine (adrenaline) and norepinephrine (noradrenaline), that enhances rapid activation of our reflex response system.

These chemicals cause an increase in heart rate, muscle tension, and blood pressure. Blood flow is diverted from the internal organs and skin, and sent to the brain and muscles. Our rate of breathing increases, our pupils dilate, and perspiration increases. The hypothalamus, interpreting the above reactions, relays information to the molecule corticotrophin-releasing hormone (CRH) as well as to other hormones. These hormones then signal the pituitary gland to release adrenocorticotrophin (ACTH) as well as other hormones in order to evoke additional adaptive responses. These adaptive responses include the release of cortisol which aids in mobilizing energy, increasing cardiovascular and cardiopulmonary activity, sharpening cognitive abilities to increase performance, and decrease the activity of the immune and digestive systems.

After you've fought, fled or otherwise escaped your stressful situation, the parasympathetic nervous system is signaled to reverse the above process bringing the body back to a "resting" state as the levels of cortisol and adrenaline in your bloodstream decline. As a result, your heart rate and blood pressure return to normal and your digestion and metabolism resume their regular pace. This entire process involves a circular informational loop between the limbic system, hypothalamus, pituitary system, and the adrenals of the body, and back again.

## The Autonomic Nervous System and the Fight Or Flight Response

| Parasympathetic System | Sympathetic System |
|---|---|
| Constricts Pupil | Dilates pupil |
| Stimulates salivation | Inhibits salivation |
| Slows heartbeat | Accelerates heartbeat |
| Slows breathing | Accelerates breathing |
| Stimulates digestion | Inhibits digestion |
| Inhibits hormones | Activates secretion of hormones |
| Contracts bladder | Relaxes bladder |
| Relaxes rectum | Contracts rectum |

*What triggers the stress response*

First, it is essential to understand that the body-mind does not know the difference between a real and imagined threat, for example; you are watching a frightening movie. Even though you may be sitting comfortably in your living room, and reason tells you that you are not actually in danger, your body still responds. When you see frightening images the brain interprets these as a danger or threat to the well being of the body, and in turn activates the fight or flight response. Your heart beat increases, your breathing quickens and becomes more shallow, your palms may become sweaty, and you may even physically jump or become startled. While at a much lower level this same set of reactions can occur due to a constant stream of negative thoughts or during periods of constant worry. These thoughts and worries are signals to the brain that something is wrong or that there is a threat to your well being, causing the body-mind to respond. This reaction can occur even if the thoughts we are having are merely anticipations about what might happen. Frequently our worries are about events that have not actually happened.

## *How does stress affect your health*

As explained above, the human body is designed to experience stress and to react to it. Stress can be positive, keeping us alert and ready to avoid danger. Stress becomes negative when a person faces continual challenges without relief or relaxation between challenges. When stressful situations pile up one after another, your body has no chance to recover. As a result, one may tend to become overworked as stress-related tension builds. Stress that continues without relief can lead to physical symptoms including headaches, upset stomach, elevated blood pressure, chest pain, and problems sleeping. The long-term activation of the stress-response system can disrupt almost all your body's processes, increasing your risk of obesity, insomnia, digestive complaints, heart disease, and depression. Research suggests that stress can also bring on or worsen certain symptoms or diseases.

Consider the following:
- Stress is linked to six of the leading causes of death: heart disease, cancer, lung ailments, accidents, cirrhosis of the liver, and suicide.
- Chronic stress can wear down the body's natural defenses and cause health problems or make problems worse if you don't learn ways to deal with it.

Stress can effect such systems of the body as:
- Digestive system. It's common to have a stomachache or diarrhea when you're stressed. This happens because stress hormones slow the release of stomach acid and the emptying of the stomach. The same hormones also stimulate the colon, which speeds the passage of its contents. Chronic stress can also lead to continuously high levels of cortisol. This hormone can increase appetite and cause weight gain.
- Immune system. Chronic stress tends to decrease the activity of your immune system, making you more susceptible to colds and other infections. Normally, your immune system responds to infection by releasing several substances that cause inflammation. In response, the adrenal glands produce cortisol, which switches off the immune and inflammatory responses once the infection is cleared. However, prolonged stress keeps your cortisol levels continuously elevated, so your immune system remains suppressed.

  In some cases, stress can have the opposite effect, making your immune system overactive. The result is an increased risk of autoimmune diseases where your immune system attacks your body's own cells. Stress can also worsen the symptoms of autoimmune diseases.
- Nervous system. If your fight-or-flight response never shuts off, stress hormones produce persistent feelings of anxiety, helplessness and impending doom. Oversensitivity to stress has

been linked with severe depression, possibly because depressed people have a harder time adapting to the negative effects of cortisol. The byproducts of cortisol act as sedatives, which contribute to the overall feeling of depression. Excessive amounts of cortisol can cause sleep disturbances, a lessening of the sex drive and loss of appetite.
- Cardiovascular system. High levels of cortisol can also raise your heart rate and increase your blood pressure and blood lipid (cholesterol and triglyceride) levels. These are risk factors for both heart attacks and strokes. Cortisol levels also appear to play a role in the accumulation of abdominal fat, which gives some people an "apple" shape. People with apple body shapes have a higher risk of heart disease and diabetes than do people with "pear" body shapes, where weight is more concentrated in the hips.
- Other systems. Stress may worsen such skin conditions as psoriasis, eczema, hives and acne, and it can be a trigger for asthma attacks.

## *Signs and symptoms of stress*

| *Physical* | *Behavioral* | *Emotional* |
|---|---|---|
| Headaches | Restlessness | Crying |
| Indigestion | Being overly critical of others | Nervousness |
| Stomach aches | Grinding one's teeth at night | Anxiety |
| Sweaty palms | Inability to get things done or make decisions | Boredom (there's no meaning to anything) |
| Hypertension (high blood pressure) | Easily upset | Edginess (a readiness to explode) |
| Dizziness or a general feeling of "being out of it" | Excessive anger and hostility | Feeling powerless to change things |
| Tension in the back, neck, face, and shoulders | Lack of creativity | An overwhelming sense of pressure |
| Heart irregularities | Problems with relationships | Loneliness |
| Insomnia | | Depression |
| Tiredness | | Constant worry |
| Trembling/shaking | | Loss of sense of humor |
| Constipation or diarrhea | | |
| Shortness of breath | | |

*Stress and Osteoporosis*

Stress management is essential in the effective management of osteoporosis because some symptoms of osteoporosis (back pain, mood swings, and hot flashes) can get worse under stress. The right amount of rest along with a regular program of stress management is a very important part of controlling the symptoms of osteoporosis. Research suggests that a regular practice of relaxation techniques may help to control the number, duration and intensity of hot flashes.

*Techniques to reduce and manage stress*

- Learn to recognize when you're feeling stressed and become conscious of your reaction to the stress.
- Choose a way to deal with your stress.
  If possible avoid the event or situation that leads to your stress. Identify areas of your life you can change to eliminate or reduce exposure to stress.
  To the best of your ability prepare for events you know may be stressful (a job interview or doctor's appointment).
- If you can not avoid the situation, change how you react to stress.
  Try to look at change as a positive challenge, not a threat. Step back from the conflict or worry and shift your outlook. Many times, simply choosing to look at situations in a more positive way can reduce the amount of stress in your life.
- Don't worry about things you can't control (the weather or other's actions).
- Teach yourself to control your physical reactions to stress.
- Build up your emotional ability to deal with stress.
- Ask for help from friends, family or professionals.
  Take a break, talk to someone close and get a different perspective on your troubles. Work to resolve conflicts with other people. On your own, you may have limited success trying to change the habitual patterns of thought and behavior that trigger your stress response. Psychiatrists, psychologists, and licensed clinical social workers are trained to help you break free of these patterns. The most important step you can take is to seek help as soon as you feel less able to cope. Taking action early will enable you to understand and deal with the many effects of osteoporosis.
- Set realistic goals at home and at work.
- Exercise on a regular basis. Exercise increases your physical capacity to deal with stress.
- Eat well-balanced meals and get enough sleep.
- Get away from your daily stresses by participating in group sports, social events, and hobbies.
- Take control. Exercise, join a support group, look outside yourself, help others.
  Talking with others in an osteoporosis support group helps you connect with people who understand what you are coping with. Find out as much as you can about the illness. Talk to your friends and family about it. Do not isolate them. They will want to be involved in helping you.
- Do things you enjoy.
- Meditate or practice relaxation techniques.

Stress management requires continuous practice as you go through life and deal with change — which often comes unexpectedly. Even if you take everyday frustrations in stride, your stress response can still surge up when you find yourself dealing with something big, such as illness, job loss, or bereavement.

*How practicing meditation and relaxation techniques can help*

Meditation and relaxation techniques are forms of focused concentration that work by introducing calm, peaceful images in the mind, creating a "mental escape." Meditation techniques provide a powerful psychological strategy that enhances a person's coping skills. Many people dealing with stress feel loss of control, fear, panic, anxiety, helplessness, and uncertainty. Research has shown that practicing meditation and relaxation techniques can help people overcome stress, anger, pain, depression, insomnia, and other problems associated with illnesses and medical/surgical procedures. Stress and depression can worsen the symptoms of osteoporosis. Meditation and relaxation techniques help you to remain calm. In addition to reducing stress and depression, meditation and relaxation techniques can:

- Dramatically decrease pain and the need for pain medication
- Decrease side effects and complications of medical procedures
- Shorten hospital stays and reduce recovery time
- Enhance sleep
- Strengthen the immune system and enhance the ability to heal
- Increase self-confidence and self-control

# Meditation/Relaxation Techniques

There are many types of meditation or relaxation techniques. All aim for the same outcome they simply utilize different techniques. Experiment with the different techniques in order to find one that works well for you. You may also find that some techniques work best in certain circumstances.

## *Basic meditation/relaxation*

When practicing this basic technique the physiological and psychological reactions that occur in the body are the exact opposite of those which happen during the activation of the fight or flight response. By regularly eliciting this calmer state, one may be able to counteract the detrimental effects of constant stress. When the fight or flight response is activated several reactions occur. These include an increase in heart rate, blood pressure, rate of respiration, muscular tension, and blood flow being directed away from the process of digestion and instead directed towards the muscles and brain. When the basic meditation exercise is practiced the exact opposite can occur. There may be a reduction in heart rate, rate of respiration, muscular tension, and an overall decrease in the body's metabolism.

## *Basic meditation technique*

The goal of the basic meditation exercise is to allow the mind to shift away from the constant stream of thoughts and worries and instead focus solely on the movement of the breath. This helps to slow down the activity and chatter in the mind, which in turn will send signals to the body-mind that you are relaxed and there is nothing to worry about. As the body-mind receives these calming signals, the brain will signal the body to calm the nervous system and reverse the effects of the fight or flight syndrome. You may also find that after meditating you may be less likely to rush around and more inclined to remain in the peaceful state you achieved during your relaxation session.

*Basic Meditation Steps*

1) Find a quiet place where you will not be disturbed for about 15-20 minutes. Turn off phones and remove as many distractions as possible.

2) Find a comfortable position that you can remain in for about 15-20 minutes. This can be sitting in a chair with the back straight but not rigid and feet flat on the floor, or sitting cross-legged on the floor. If you find sitting cross-legged on the floor uncomfortable on your knees or back, you can sit on a cushion or pillow in order to raise your hips a bit higher then your knees. This will help to both take pressure off of the knees and maintain a straight back. You can also lie down for this exercise, as long as you do not fall asleep.

3) Close the eyes and begin to focus on your breath.
Inhale through the nose and allow your abdominal area to rise, as if you were filling this area with air. Exhale through the nose and allow the stomach to fall as the air leaves this area. Sometimes it is easier to start with the exhalation and just once, contract the abdominal muscles and push the air out. Then allow the stomach to relax and rise with the inhalation. It is normal for this style of breathing to feel backwards or awkward at first but with practice it will become easier.

For the next 20 minutes remain focused on your breath. To keep the mind focused allow yourself to be aware of the abdomen as it rises and falls, or allow your attention to remain on the sensation of the air as it enters and exits the nose. If these sensations are difficult to focus on, the breath can be counted by silently saying one on the inhale and two on the exhale. If the mind does wander, which it will, simply without judgment bring your attention back to the breath.

When first attempting this exercise you may need to bring your attention back quite often. However, keeping your attention on the breath and away from other thoughts will become easier with practice. You can time yourself for the 20 minutes, however, avoid using a loud alarm as you do not want to startle the body out of meditation. An alarm which can be programmed to come on with soft music could be used. You could choose to play soft music for 15 to 20 minutes as a way to time yourself. It is not recommended to continually open the eyes and look at the time as this disrupts the process of concentrated meditation. When the 20 minutes is up, allow yourself time and do not get up too quickly. Take a few minutes to feel the results of your meditation.

4) Remember to keep a passive attitude. Meditation is a skill and like any new skill, takes practice. Remember to not get concerned about doing the exercise correctly and be careful about expecting any particular results. The object is to simply take time out of the day to give the body-mind a break from everyday thoughts and worries.

*Note:*
 The breathing is taught in and out of the nose, since this is physiologically more relaxing for the body. However if you are experiencing respiratory or sinus issues and find this difficult you can breathe through the mouth. You may find that with practice, breathing strictly through the nose will become easier.

## Autogenic Training (AT)

This technique trains the body-mind to become quiet and relaxed by utilizing self-suggestions. These self-suggestions attempt to change the thoughts present in the mind, by suggesting to the body-mind that certain events are occurring. These events can include a slower heartbeat, increased blood flow, and less muscle tension. Since research suggests the possibility that negative thoughts can result in decreased efficiency of the systems in the body, advocates of AT suggest that we can utilize positive thoughts to enhance the efficiency of the systems of the body.

### *Autogenic Training exercise*
If you find that these particular suggestions do not apply to your situation, please feel free to substitute any other "suggestions." You may wish to record these instructions onto a tape until you are more familiar with the process.

Find a comfortable position which you can remain in for about 20 minutes where you will not be disturbed. Begin to focus on your breath and allow your body to relax. Slowly and silently count down from four to one. When you reach the number 1 you will be completely relaxed.

Concentrate on your right arm. Slowly and silently say to yourself six times, my right arm is very heavy.
Concentrate on your left arm. Slowly and silently say to yourself six times, my left arm is very heavy.
Concentrate on both arms. Slowly and silently say to yourself six times, my arms are very heavy.
Turn your attention away from your arms, and silently say to yourself just once, I am very quiet, and I enjoy feeling relaxed for a while.

Concentrate on your right leg. Slowly and silently say to yourself six times, my right leg is very heavy.
Concentrate on your left leg. Slowly and silently say to yourself six times my left leg is very heavy.
Concentrate on both legs. Slowly and silently say to yourself six times my legs are very heavy.
Turn your attention away from your legs, and silently say to yourself just once, I am very quiet, and I enjoy feeling relaxed for a while.

Concentrate on the beating of your heart. Slowly and silently say to yourself six times, my heartbeat is calm and strong.
Turn your attention away from your heartbeat, and silently say to yourself just once, I am very quiet and I enjoy feeling relaxed for a while.

Concentrate on the rhythm of your breathing. Slowly and silently say to yourself six times, my breathing is slow and deep.
Turn your attention away from your breath and silently say to yourself just once, I am very quiet and I enjoy feeling relaxed for a while.

Concentrate on your stomach. Slowly and silently say to yourself six times, warmth is radiating throughout my stomach and throughout my body.
Turn your attention away from your stomach and silently say to yourself just once, I am very quiet and I enjoy feeling relaxed, for a while.

Concentrate on your forehead. Slowly and silently say to yourself six times, my forehead is cool.
Turn your attention away from your forehead and silently say to yourself just once, I am very quiet and I enjoy feeling relaxed, for a while.

Bring your attention back to your breath.
Slowly and silently count down from four to one. By the time you reach the number one, you will be alert and awake, yet relaxed.

Begin to circle the wrists and ankles, gently stretching and moving the body. When you are ready, slowly open the eyes. Take a few minutes to feel the effects of your meditation.

# Guided Imagery

Where Autogenic Training utilizes self-suggestion, guided imagery relies on images to suggest physiological changes to the body-mind creating harmony between the mind and body. Guided imagery or visualization is a process by which you create calm, peaceful images in your mind in order to help elicit a state of relaxation or manage symptoms. Guided imagery, much like the basic meditation exercise, aims to present the brain with different stimuli to focus on, allowing for a break from everyday thoughts and worries. Imagery is often used to stimulate changes in bodily functions that are usually considered inaccessible to conscious influence. Imagery can be effective, as research suggests that the brain will respond to mentally created images much in the same way it responds to actually seeing images. A common example of how this works is to try the following exercise.

*First try to imagine a lemon... Use all of your senses... Smell the lemon and get a sense of its texture... Next, recall what a lemon tastes like... Now imagine cutting open the lemon and squirting some of the lemon juice into your mouth... Imagine swishing the lemon juice around in your mouth and then swallowing it.*

In this exercise even though tasting the lemon was only in your imagination you may have noticed changes in your body. You might have begun to salivate and you might have even puckered at the thought of the taste. In this example your body-mind responded to the thought as though the event actually took place. Constant worry is another example of the effects of imagery. As you worry about events that may or may not happen, your body-mind may respond by tensing muscles and arousing the nervous system in anticipation of a challenge.

Imagery can also provide a way to communicate conscious intentions or requests to your unconscious mind. When using guided imagery the participant might visualize a scene such as a beach, meadow, or other such place which can elicit feelings of relaxation and peace. In this example when imagining such a scene, the body-mind receives signals that it is all right to relax since there is no threat present. Imagery may also be used when dealing with a particular disease such as cancer. In this case the patient may use imagery to visualize the body-mind healing itself from the disease by "seeing" or imagining their immune system eliminating the cancerous cells. Imagery, like many of the complementary techniques available can be used in conjunction with medical treatment. For someone who is taking medication for an illness, imagery could be used to visualize the treatment working. As with most all forms of meditation, the practice of guided imagery or visualization can help to interrupt the flow of constant thoughts and worries, and thereby allow the body-mind to rest, conserve energy, and build energy reserves.

Using guided imagery (or other types of meditation) to manage stress and symptoms can provide a sense of hope and encourage feelings of control over one's situation. However, as with any form of meditation, a passive attitude is essential. While it is important to make the images as real as possible, it is just as important to not focus on results or particular outcomes. When an end result or outcome is the focus, anxiety and tension can result which are counterproductive to stress and symptom management.

When first practicing guided imagery it may seem difficult to actually "see" the images. It is important to know that with practice, visualizing images will become easier. It is important to not become frustrated or tense if visualization exercises do not come easily. Sometimes it may be easier to "sense" the image versus struggling to "see" the image. For example if trying to visualize a healing light, instead of "seeing" the light you may choose to just "sense" that it is there, by focusing on a sensation of warmth or heat, a tingling sensation, or just simply knowing that it is there.

You can also practice improving your guided imagery ability with a simple exercise. First notice a basic object around your home. Make it something simple without a lot of design. Observe the object for a few minutes and really notice its detail. Then, close your eyes and try to recall the object in your mind's eye. Recall the shape, size, color, smell, texture etc. Try this with various objects keeping it simple at first, and then work up to more detailed objects.

### *Guided Imagery/Visualization Exercise.*

There are many different versions of imagery exercises, however the example below is a commonly used technique. It will be easier to either record the instructions on a tape or have someone read them to you so you can remain focused on the process versus continually having to stop and look at the directions. As with the basic meditation exercise, find a way to time yourself so you are not startled out of the meditation. You will need approximately twenty minutes for this exercise.

1) Begin by practicing the basic meditation technique for approximately five to ten minutes. The time does not need to be exact, but it should be long enough for you to feel a shift in the state of tension and relaxation of your body.
The following is the script to use for the imagery section. Where I have included "….." signals a time to give yourself a few minutes in-between the next instruction.

2) Begin to imagine yourself walking on a private beach on a perfect summer day………
Take some time to look around and use all of your senses to explore the area………
Hear the waves as they come up gently on the shore……….
Feel the warm sun on your skin and the sand underneath your feet…………
Smell the salt air……….. notice how being here makes you feel……………

Find a place where you can sit or lie down either on the shore, in the water, or anywhere else that looks inviting to you…………..
Begin to become aware of the light and warmth from the sun…………
As you relax here allow this warmth and light to permeate your skin and be absorbed into the body………
Allow yourself to imagine this light and warmth to have healing properties………….
If there are any areas of tightness, tension, or disease present in the body-mind allow these things to be dissolved by the warmth and light…………….
Take some time here to relax and heal the body-mind……………
 (allow 10-15 min. here for this experience)

Begin to bring your attention back to the breath…………….
Feel the abdomen rise as you inhale and the abdomen fall as you exhale………
Allow yourself to slowly and gently become a little more awake and a little more alert with each breath…………..become aware of the pressures against your body from the floor or chair………..
Then when you are ready slowly open the eyes.

3) Allow yourself to come out of the meditation slowly and take some time to feel the effects of the exercise.

4) Remember to maintain a passive attitude. Visualizing images can be difficult at first, however, it will become easier with practice. If you find visualizing the above difficult, you can try to focus on sensation instead. In this example, you would allow yourself to feel the sensation of being at a relaxed spot, and focus more on the sensation of the warmth of the sun entering your body versus focusing on actually visualizing the light.

## Mindfulness Meditation

This form of meditation, which has its roots in Buddhism, is focused on learning to become fully present in the moment and to be fully accepting of whatever is occurring in the present moment. Unlike the three other forms of meditation presented, this form of meditation aims to help the participant change their response to stimuli rather then alter their physiology. The goal is for the meditator to be fully aware of the stimuli around them, (such as noise or other people), yet learn to not react to the stimuli. This process is also referred to as learning to become a dispassionate watcher or a witness. During this process the participant aims to become aware of the mind's constant stream of thoughts and to it's constant judgement and reaction to inner and outer experiences. This technique aims to teach you how to not get caught up in these thoughts by allowing yourself to step back from the thoughts.

An example of this would be meditating while experiencing pain. In the basic meditation exercise, the participant tries to interrupt the pain signals, and the typical anxiety laden thoughts that accompany them, by shifting the mind's attention onto awareness of the breath, since interrupting the flow of thoughts can often aid in reducing symptoms. Autogenic Training would utilize self-suggestions such as the area which is painful, is becoming more relaxed and is therefore more comfortable. In the case of guided imagery the participant might try mentally visualizing the pain as a red ball which then turns into a softer color and becomes smaller and smaller until the ball disappears. With these types of meditation the aim is to interrupt the stream of thoughts which are occurring in the mind, but also suggest to the body-mind that the pain no longer exists.

However, when using mindfulness meditation, the participant would not attempt any of the above. Rather the meditator would acknowledge the pain but attempt to not react to it with thoughts of anger, depression or frustration. Approaching the sensation of pain in this way gives the body-mind an alternate way of seeing discomfort. Instead of becoming agitated by the sensation the meditator would relate to the experience or sensation of pain simply as an event that is happening in the present, but would refrain from allowing the mind to wander to negative thoughts about the sensation. In other words the meditator would not allow the mind to become distracted with thoughts which attempt to predict what the pain may or may not do in the future, or how the pain effects their life. This process attempts to run interference so that thoughts, emotions and/or memories do not integrate the experience of pain with the activation of the fight or flight response. This form of meditation can help the participant to learn to lessen the times the body-mind is activated when exposed to stress.

The limbic system (the emotional center of the brain) is directly linked to the hypothalamus region which aids in the regulation of the autonomic nervous system. By learning to not allow emotions to take charge (getting angry about the pain) the hypothalamus in turn does not receive the signal to activate the stress response. This form of meditation is based on a fundamental Buddhist belief - that the origin of much of our suffering comes from a constant need to grasp onto things and the attempt to change what is.

## *Mindfulness Meditation Exercise*

Below is a sample of a typical mindfulness meditation exercise. As with the other forms of meditation, find a way to time yourself for twenty minutes so you will not be startled out of the exercise.

1) Begin by practicing the basic meditation technique for approximately five to ten minutes. The time does not need to be exact, but it should be long enough for you to feel a shift in the state of tension and relaxation of your body.

2) When your body-mind has quieted down, try shifting your awareness to the process of thinking and take your attention off of the breath. Attempt to be a dispassionate observer as you simply "watch" the thoughts that come into your mind. Try to perceive the thoughts simply as events in your mind. Try to not allow yourself to become caught up in the thoughts, just notice that they are there. Notice their content and the rate at which they change. Notice that each particular thought does not last very long, but rather individual thoughts come and go, and sometimes the same thought will keep coming back. If you notice sensations of discomfort, allow yourself to become aware of the sensations, yet choose to not react to them. Notice if the sensations change with time. Again try to practice being the observer of an event. Notice if by simply observing the sensation you can allow yourself to become detached from the sensation. (However if you are experiencing significant discomfort do not force yourself to continue with this exercise).
To end the meditation bring your awareness back to your breathing for a few minutes.

3) End the meditation slowly and allow yourself a few minutes to experience the effects of this exercise.

4) Remember to maintain a passive attitude. Try to avoid getting caught up in how well you performed the meditation or becoming attached to any particular results.

This form of meditation can be challenging at first. You may find it difficult to stay with this exercise for a full 20 minutes. If this occurs, start by practicing for just a few minutes at a time and slowly build up to a 15-20 minute practice.

# Resource Section

This book has covered many techniques and forms of movement, which can help in managing the symptoms and challenges faced by those with osteoporosis. In addition, there are many other opinions, approaches, and techniques not covered in this book. We encourage you to explore all of the options available and try many different approaches. With exploration you will find the approach that works best for your unique situation.

This section will provide sample routines, workout logs, and suggestions for using the information in this book. These are provided as a guide only to help you in getting started in developing your own routine. As you learn how different movements affect you, you can then work to develop your own routine.

For the best results, you need to do some exercise everyday. You do not need to do all of the exercises in this book every day. It is best to alter your routine between a variety of exercises. Doing the same exact workout every time you exercise, will cause the body to adapt to the routine and lessen the affect of the exercise. To keep the body responding to exercise it is important to periodically change your routine or change the amount or type of resistance you are using.

- Things you should try to do everyday include:
  1. Deep diaphragmatic breathing exercises. Try for 10-15 minutes of deep breathing each day.
  2. Stretching to bring the shoulders back and open the chest.
  3. Balancing exercises.
  4. Relaxation technique.
  5. Some type of weight bearing activity

- Things you should do at least two to three times per week.
  1. Aerobic or cardiovascular exercise that is *weight bearing*. This can either be the aerobic exercises from chapter two or walking. During the week you can alternate the aerobic exercises with a brisk 15-30 minute walk. You should walk at a pace that gets your heart rate up and you should feel slightly out of breath. Make sure you use correct walking form (pg. 27) using heel-toe walking and swing your arms (opposite arm to leg). An indicator of good cardiovascular health is being able to complete a 15-minute mile. This may be too fast of a pace, but gives you something to aim for.
  2. Strengthening exercises for the arms, legs, and abdominal muscles.
  3. A full body stretching routine.

At least once per week, get down on the floor and practice getting back up (pg. 40). Keep yourself in practice of getting up and down off of the floor. Then if you should fall you will know how to get up without having to wait for assistance.

# Sample Weekly Routine 1

You do not need to do the exercises all at the same time, they can be done throughout the day. Remember, the following routines are "the ideal" involving some exercise every day. There may be times when you miss your workout or are not feeling up to exercise, or are only able to do part of it. Use your own judgment as to what is best for your body, and how much exercise is appropriate. Make a commitment to exercise as often as you realistically can and be gentle with your body when needed. These routines take approximately one hour per day.

*Monday*
Aerobic exercises.
Strength training exercises.
10-15 minutes of deep breathing and meditation technique.

*Tuesday*
Walk for 15-20 minutes or to tolerance.
Yoga exercises.
10-15 minutes of deep breathing and meditation technique.

*Wednesday*
Aerobic exercises.
Strength training exercises.
10-15 minutes of deep breathing and meditation technique.

*Thursday*
Walk for 15-20 minutes or to tolerance.
T'ai Chi exercises.
10-15 minutes of deep breathing and meditation technique.

*Friday*
Aerobic exercises.
Strength training exercises.
10-15 minutes of deep breathing and meditation technique.

*Saturday*
Some type of aerobic exercise different from walking or the aerobic exercises in this book. Examples include swimming, water walking, or some sport you enjoy.
10-15 minutes of deep breathing and meditation technique.

*Sunday*
Pick an activity you enjoy to get the body moving and challenge your balance.

# Sample Weekly Routine 2

*Monday*
Aerobic exercises.
Upper body strength training exercises.
10-15 minutes of deep breathing and meditation technique.

*Tuesday*
Walk for 15-20 minutes or to tolerance.
Lower body strength training exercises.
Yoga exercises.
10-15 minutes of deep breathing and meditation technique.

*Wednesday*
Aerobic exercises.
Upper body strength training exercises.
10-15 minutes of deep breathing and meditation technique.

*Thursday*
Walk for 15-20 minutes or to tolerance.
Lower body strength training exercises.
T'ai Chi exercises.
10-15 minutes of deep breathing and meditation technique.

*Friday*
Aerobic exercises.
Upper body strength training exercises.
10-15 minutes of deep breathing and meditation technique.

*Saturday*
Some type of aerobic exercise different from walking or the aerobic exercises in this book. Examples include swimming, water walking, or some sport you enjoy.
10-15 minutes of deep breathing and meditation technique.

*Sunday*
Pick an activity you enjoy to get the body moving and challenge your balance.
10-15 minutes of deep breathing and meditation technique.

# Workout Logs

You can use these logs to keep track of your progress for the aerobic and strength training exercises. Keeping a record of your workouts helps you to stay on track and can help motivate you to continue as you see the increase in your exercise tolerance.

In the boxes mark down the amount of time you competed each exercise. There are blank boxes provided to write in your own activities.

## SAMPLE
### *Aerobic exercise log*

Week of _01___/_05___/_04___

|  | Sun. | Mon. | Tues. | Wed. | Thurs. | Fri. | Sat. |
|---|---|---|---|---|---|---|---|
| March in place |  | 1 min. |  | 2 min. |  | 1 min. |  |
| Straight leg kick |  | 1 min. |  | 2 min. |  | 1 min. |  |
| Step side to side |  | 1 min. |  | 2 min. |  | 1 min. |  |
| Knee lifts |  | 1 min. |  | 2 min. |  | 1 min. |  |
| Heel curls back |  | 1 min. |  | 2 min. |  | 1 min. |  |
| Side toe taps |  | 1 min. |  | 2 min. |  | 1 min. |  |
| Heel taps |  | 1 min. |  | 2 min. |  | 1 min. |  |
| Walking |  |  | 20 min. |  | 15 min. |  | 20 min. |
| Swimming | 20 min. |  |  |  |  |  |  |
|  |  |  |  |  |  |  |  |
|  |  |  |  |  |  |  |  |

*Aerobic exercise log*

*Week of* \_\_\_\_/\_\_\_\_/\_\_\_\_

|  | Sun. | Mon. | Tues. | Wed. | Thurs. | Fri. | Sat. |
|---|---|---|---|---|---|---|---|
| March in place |  |  |  |  |  |  |  |
| Straight leg kick |  |  |  |  |  |  |  |
| Step side to side |  |  |  |  |  |  |  |
| Knee lifts |  |  |  |  |  |  |  |
| Heel curls back |  |  |  |  |  |  |  |
| Side toe taps |  |  |  |  |  |  |  |
| Heel taps |  |  |  |  |  |  |  |
| Walking |  |  |  |  |  |  |  |
|  |  |  |  |  |  |  |  |
|  |  |  |  |  |  |  |  |
|  |  |  |  |  |  |  |  |

# SAMPLE
## *Strength training log*
### Week of __01__/__05__/__04__

|  | Sun. | Mon. | Tues. | Wed. | Thurs. | Fri. | Sat. |
|---|---|---|---|---|---|---|---|
| Leg extension |  | 10 reps<br>3 pounds |  | 10 reps<br>3 pounds |  | 10 reps<br>3 pounds |  |
| Squat |  | 10 reps |  | 10 reps |  | 10 reps |  |
| Side leg lift |  | 10 reps<br>3 pounds |  | 10 reps<br>3 pounds |  | 10 reps<br>3 pounds |  |
| Leg lift back |  | 10 reps<br>3 pounds |  | 10 reps<br>3 pounds |  | 10 reps<br>3 pounds |  |
| Heel curl |  | 10 reps<br>3 pounds |  | 10 reps<br>3 pounds |  | 10 reps<br>3 pounds |  |
| Leg crossover |  | 10 reps<br>3 pounds |  | 10 reps<br>3 pounds |  | 10 reps<br>3 pounds |  |
| Heel raises |  | 10 reps<br>3 pounds |  | 10 reps<br>3 pounds |  | 10 reps<br>3 pounds |  |
| Toe raises |  | 10 reps<br>3 pounds |  | 10 reps<br>3 pounds |  | 10 reps<br>3 pounds |  |
| Wall pushups |  |  | 12 reps |  | 12 reps |  | 12 reps |
| Bent row |  |  | 10 reps<br>2 pounds |  | 10 reps<br>2 pounds |  | 10 reps<br>2 pounds |
| Military press |  |  | 10 reps<br>2 pounds |  | 10 reps<br>2 pounds |  | 10 reps<br>2 pounds |
| Deltoid raise |  |  | 10 reps<br>2 pounds |  | 10 reps<br>2 pounds |  | 10 reps<br>2 pounds |
| Biceps curl |  |  | 10 reps<br>2 pounds |  | 10 reps<br>2 pounds |  | 10 reps<br>2 pounds |
| Triceps kickback |  |  | 10 reps<br>2 pounds |  | 10 reps<br>2 pounds |  | 10 reps<br>2 pounds |
| Wrist curls |  |  | 10 reps<br>2 pounds |  | 10 reps<br>2 pounds |  | 10 reps<br>2 pounds |
| Reverse wrist curls |  |  | 10 reps<br>2 pounds |  | 10 reps<br>2 pounds |  | 10 reps<br>2 pounds |
| Lean backs |  | 12 reps |  | 12 reps |  | 12 reps |  |
| Side bends |  | 10 reps<br>2 pounds |  | 10 reps<br>2 pounds |  | 10 reps<br>2 pounds |  |

*Strength training log*
*Week of* \_\_\_\_/\_\_\_\_/\_\_\_\_

|  | Sun. | Mon. | Tues. | Wed. | Thurs. | Fri. | Sat. |
|---|---|---|---|---|---|---|---|
| Leg extension | | | | | | | |
| Squat | | | | | | | |
| Side leg lift | | | | | | | |
| Leg lift back | | | | | | | |
| Heel curl | | | | | | | |
| Leg crossover | | | | | | | |
| Heel raises | | | | | | | |
| Toe raises | | | | | | | |
| Wall pushups | | | | | | | |
| Bent row | | | | | | | |
| Military press | | | | | | | |
| Deltoid raise | | | | | | | |
| Biceps curl | | | | | | | |
| Triceps kickback | | | | | | | |
| Wrist curls | | | | | | | |
| Reverse wrist curls | | | | | | | |
| Lean backs | | | | | | | |
| Side bends | | | | | | | |

## *Yoga Log*
### *Week of  ____/____/____*

|  | Sun. | Mon. | Tues. | Wed. | Thurs. | Fri. | Sat. |
|---|---|---|---|---|---|---|---|
| Head rotation/stretch | | | | | | | |
| Neck rolls/stretch | | | | | | | |
| Shoulder rolls | | | | | | | |
| Shoulder strap stretches | | | | | | | |
| Chin tuck | | | | | | | |
| Chest opener | | | | | | | |
| Cat stretch | | | | | | | |
| Ankle exercises | | | | | | | |
| Mountain pose | | | | | | | |
| Warrior I | | | | | | | |
| Warrior II | | | | | | | |
| Lateral angle | | | | | | | |
| Standing half moon | | | | | | | |
| Chair pose | | | | | | | |
| Salute to the sun | | | | | | | |
| Tree pose | | | | | | | |
| Warrior III | | | | | | | |
| Dancer's pose | | | | | | | |
| Victory squat | | | | | | | |
| Chest stretch | | | | | | | |
| Hamstring stretch | | | | | | | |
| Pelvic tilts | | | | | | | |
| Bridge | | | | | | | |
| Knee to chest | | | | | | | |
| Spinal twist | | | | | | | |
| Singe arm and leg raises | | | | | | | |
| Opposite arm to leg raises | | | | | | | |
| Boat pose | | | | | | | |
| Spinx pose | | | | | | | |
| Cat pose | | | | | | | |
| Leg strap stretches | | | | | | | |
| Child pose | | | | | | | |
| Bound angle pose | | | | | | | |

## Tai Chi Log
### Week of ____/____/____

| | Sun. | Mon. | Tues. | Wed. | Thurs. | Fri. | Sat. |
|---|---|---|---|---|---|---|---|
| Press energy down | | | | | | | |
| Spread eagle's wings | | | | | | | |
| Gather energy | | | | | | | |
| Waist twists | | | | | | | |
| Waist bends | | | | | | | |
| T'ai chi walk | | | | | | | |
| Chasing clouds | | | | | | | |
| Tandem walk | | | | | | | |

# Diary for Stress Management/Meditation Exercises

Many of our clients have found it helpful to keep diaries or journals as part of their stress management program. Below is a sample page we use in our program. You can use one sheet for each time you practice or you may wish to write in a diary or journal.

Technique Used _____

Time of day you practiced _____

Length of time you practiced _____

How did you feel before your practice?

_____

_____

How did you feel after your practice?

_____

_____

List any experiences which you decided to respond to differently than you usually would.

_____

_____

# Helpful Organizations and Webpages

*Information on Osteoporosis (Treatment, education, research and services)*

National Osteoporosis Foundation
1232 22nd Street N.W.
Washington, D.C. 20037-1292
Phone: (202) 223.2226
www.nof.org

Office of the Surgeon General
5600 Fishers Lane
Room 18-66
Rockville, MD 20857
Bone Health and Osteoporosis: A Report of the Surgeon General
Issued October 14, 2004
www.surgeongeneral.gov/library/bonehealth/

Foundation for Osteoporosis Research and Education
300 27th Street, Suite 103
Oakland, CA 94612
Phone: Toll free (888) 266-3015
www.fore.org

The International Osteoporosis Foundation
Swiss office:
5 Rue Perdtemps
1260 Nyon
Switzerland
Phone: +41 22 994 01 00
www.osteofound.org/index.php

Nutrition Information
American Dietetic Association Headquarters
120 South Riverside Plaza, Suite 2000
Chicago, IL 60606-6995
Phone: (800) 877-1600
www.eatright.org/Public

Food and Drug Administration
5600 Fishers Lane
Rockville, Maryland 20857
Phone: (888) 463-6332
Boning Up on Osteoporosis
www.fda.gov/fdac/features/796_bone.html

***Information on fitness  (Exercise, healthy lifestyle topics, finding a qualified instructor)***

American College Of Sports Medicine
P.O. Box 1440
Indianapolis, IN 46206-1440
Phone: (317) 637-9200
www.acsm.org

National Institute of Health
9000 Rockville Pike
Bethesda, Maryland 20892
Phone: (301) 496-4000
www.nih.gov

National Institute of Aging
Building 31, Room 5C27
31 Center Drive, MSC 2292
Bethesda, MD 20892
www.nih.gov/nia

*Information on yoga (Types of yoga, postures, books, videos, tapes, finding a qualified instructor)*

Kripalu Center for Yoga and Health
P.O. Box 793
West Street, Route 183
Lenox, MA 01240
Phone: (800) 741-7353
www.kripalu.org

National Yoga Alliance
7801 Old Branch Avenue Suite 400
Clinton, MD 20735
Phone: Toll free (877) 964-2255
www.nationalyogaalliance.org

Yoga Journal
475 Sansome Street, Suite 850
San Francisco, CA 94111
Phone: (415) 591-0555,
www.yogajournal.com

Information on stress management and meditation (Forms of meditation, techniques, videos, tapes

Academy for Guided Imagery
30765 Pacific Coast Highway, Suite 369
Malibu, CA 90265
Phone: (800) 726-2070
www.academyforguidedimagery.com

Bernie Siegel/ECAP
522 Jackson Park Drive
Meadville, PA 16335
Phone: (814) 337-8192
www.ecap-online.org/

Jon Kabat-Zin
Stress Reduction Tapes
P.O. Box 547
Lexington, MA 02420
www.mindfulnesstapes.com

The Mind Body Medical Institute at Beth Israel Deaconess Hospital
824 Boylston Street
Chestnut Hill, MA 02467
Phone: (617) 991-0102
www.mbmi.com

Thich Nhat Hahn
Plum Village
www.plumvillage.org/

Umass Medical Center
The Center for Mindfulness in Medicine, Health Care, and Society
55 Lake Avenue North Worcester, MA 01655
Phone: (508) 856-2656
www.umassmed.edu/cfm/

***Information on physical therapy (How physical therapy can help, health articles finding a therapist)***

American Physical Therapy Association
1111 North Fairfax Street
Alexandria, VA 22314-1488
Phone: (800) 999-2782
www.apta.org
It is often helpful to check your local library for further resources.

# Index

## A
Abdominal exercises ............................................. 116
Aerobic exercise ..................................................... 45
Aerobic exercises ................................................... 64
Aerobic routine ...................................................... 84
Autogenic training ............................................... 221

## B
Balance; maintaining ........................................... 121
Basic meditation exercise .................................... 220
Blood pressure ....................................................... 49
Body mechanics principals .................................... 16
Bone density tests ................................................... 7

## C
Calcium .................................................................... 8
Cardiovascular system ........................................... 48

## D
Diaphragmatic breathing ........................................ 52

## E
Effects of exercise on the heart ............................. 48
Effects of exercise on the respiratory system ...... 50
Effects of meditation ........................................... 217
Effects of stress on the body ............................... 215
Exercise logs ........................................................ 231

## F
Falls; causes of .................................................... 121
Fight or flight syndrome ...................................... 213
Flexibility ............................................................. 124

## G
Getting in and out of bed ...................................... 29
Getting in and out of a car .................................... 25
Getting in and out of a chair ................................. 22
Getting up and down from the floor ..................... 40
Guided imagery ................................................... 223

## H
Heart; basic structure of ........................................ 48
Hip hinge ............................................................... 19

## L
Lifting correctly ..................................................... 37
Lungs; basic structure of ....................................... 50

## M
Making exercise part of your day ......................... 14
Managing stress ................................................... 215
Meditation diary .................................................. 237
Mindfulness meditation ....................................... 226
Music for aerobics ................................................ 47

## N
Nervous system ................................................... 213

## O
Osteoporosis ............................................................ 4

## P
Pelvic tilt ............................................................. 165

## R
Rating of perceived exertion ................................. 46
Rhythmic limbering exercises ............................... 55
Risk factors for osteoporosis .................................. 5

## S
Sitting correctly ..................................................... 21
Standing correctly ................................................. 26
Strength training .................................................... 86
Strength training exercises legs ............................. 91
Strength training arms ......................................... 105
Stress ................................................................... 212
Stress and osteoporosis ....................................... 216

## T

T'ai chi ..................................................... 195
T'ai chi walk ............................................. 207
T'ai chi warm up ...................................... 197
Talk test ..................................................... 46
Ten rep max ............................................... 87

## W

Walking correctly ...................................... 27
Web pages; helpful .................................. 239
Weight Bearing exercise ........................... 10
Workout log; aerobic .............................. 232
Workout log; strength training ............... 232

## Y

Yoga ........................................................... 84
Yoga warm up ......................................... 132
Yoga standing poses ............................... 145
Yoga floor stretches ................................ 165

For more information on our programs and products:

Living Well Yoga and Fitness
PO Box 1057
Montauk, NY 11954
(631) 259-1385
www.lwyf.org